HEALTH AT RISK

*The Columbia University Press and Social Science Research Council
Series on the Privatization of Risk*

THE COLUMBIA UNIVERSITY PRESS AND SOCIAL SCIENCE RESEARCH COUNCIL SERIES ON THE PRIVATIZATION OF RISK

Edited by Craig Calhoun and Jacob S. Hacker

The early twenty-first century is witnessing a concerted effort to privatize risk—to shift responsibility for the management or mitigation of key risks onto private-sector organizations or directly onto individuals. This series uses social science research to analyze this issue in depth. Each volume presents a concise review of a particular topic from the perspective of the public and private allocation of risk and responsibility and offers analysis and empirical, evidence-based opinion from leading scholars in the fields of economics, political science, sociology, anthropology, and law. Support for the series comes from the John D. and Catherine T. MacArthur Foundation.

Andrew Lakoff, ed., *Disaster and the Politics of Intervention*

Donald W. Light, ed., *The Risks of Prescription Drugs*

Katherine S. Newman, ed., *Laid Off, Laid Low: Political and Economic Consequences of Employment Insecurity*

Mitchell A. Orenstein, ed., *Pensions, Social Security, and the Privatization of Risk*

Health at Risk

America's Ailing Health System —
and How to Heal It

EDITED BY JACOB S. HACKER

COLUMBIA UNIVERSITY PRESS | NEW YORK

A COLUMBIA/SSRC BOOK

COLUMBIA UNIVERSITY PRESS
Publishers Since 1893
New York   Chichester, West Sussex

Copyright © 2008 Columbia University Press
All rights reserved

Library of Congress Cataloging-in-Publication Data

Health at risk : America's ailing health system—and how
to heal it / edited by Jacob S. Hacker.
     p. cm.—(The Columbia University Press
and Social Science Research Council series on the
privatization of risk)
    ISBN 978-0-231-14602-9 (cloth : alk. paper)—
    ISBN 978-0-231-14603-6 (pbk. : alk. paper)
    1. Health care reform—United States. 2. Medical
policy—United States. I. Hacker, Jacob S. II. Title.
III. Series.
    [DNLM: 1. Insurance, Health—United States.
2. Health Care Reform—United States. 3. Health
Services Accessiblity—United States. 4. Insurance
Coverage—United States. W 275 AA1 H215 2008]
RA395.A3H385 2008
362.1'04250973—dc22

                        2008020479

Columbia University Press books are printed
on permanent and durable acid-free paper. This
book is printed on paper with recycled content.
Printed in the United States of America

c 10 9 8 7 6 5 4 3 2 1
p 10 9 8 7 6 5 4 3 2

References to Internet Web sites (URLs) were
accurate at the time of writing. Neither the editor
nor Columbia University Press is responsible
for URLs that may have expired or changed since
the manuscript was prepared.

Design by Julie Fry
Cover by Vin Dang

CONTENTS

Introduction   1
JACOB S. HACKER

CHAPTER ONE
The Transformation of
American Health Insurance   10
JILL QUADAGNO &
J. BRANDON MC KELVEY

CHAPTER TWO
Uninsured in America:
New Realities, New Risks   32
KATHERINE SWARTZ

CHAPTER THREE
Get Sick, Go Broke   66
DEBORAH THORNE &
ELIZABETH WARREN

CHAPTER FOUR
Just How Good *Is*
American Medical Care?   88
ELIZABETH A. MC GLYNN,
DAVID MELTZER,
& JACOB S. HACKER

CHAPTER FIVE
The New Push for
American Health Security   106
JACOB S. HACKER

List of Contributors   138

HEALTH AT RISK

Introduction

JACOB S. HACKER

Major reform of American health insurance has once again risen to the top of the political agenda. For the past fifteen years, large-scale changes to the nation's $2.2 trillion medical complex were considered infeasible — too costly, too politically controversial, and too threatening to existing stakeholders to stand any chance of enactment. But for at least the fifth time since reformers struggled to enact compulsory health plans for workers at the state level in the 1910s, the goal of guaranteeing insurance coverage for working Americans has reignited as a burning issue.[1]

Two concerns dominate the growing public discussion: the dwindling reach and generosity of private insurance coverage, and the rapidly escalating cost of medical care. (A third concern, the uneven quality of American medical care, is rising in prominence as well.) These twin worries frequently come together in a single phrase: "health security" — protection against the potentially ruinous costs of health care and a stable foundation of access to quality medical services. Today, many Americans and their leaders believe that health security in the United States is declining and that substantial government action is required to safeguard and improve it. Yet fierce debate continues about how urgently such action is required and what form it should take.

Much of the debate is dominated by claims and counterclaims with little or no basis in serious research. Partisans on both sides make broad assertions unsupported by the facts, abuse statistical data, and misuse foreign and historical examples. In the heat of political battle, there is understandably little attention to the findings of scholarly investigations, much less careful attempt to weigh competing interpretations of the evidence. Nonetheless, the shrill charges that dominate our public discourse should not be taken to indicate that nothing firm is known about the financing, organization, and delivery of American health care, or how they could be made better. In fact, health policy experts in a range of fields have made enormous progress in understanding how America's health system operates. And they have also carefully outlined ideas both big and small for improving how this system works.

This book is an effort to bring these findings and proposals more fully into public discussion. Sponsored by the Social Science Research Council (SSRC), the world's preeminent organization advancing research in the social sciences, this volume is premised on the notion that all of us are entitled to our own opinions about American health care, but not our own facts. The pages to come carefully examine these facts, as revealed in cutting-edge social science research. Noted experts on health coverage, the quality of care, medical bankruptcy, the history of American health insurance, and the politics of health reform draw on the best existing social science research and their own expertise to speak to the pressing issues that face our nation today.

The contributors to this volume have not checked their opinions at the door. But they have all grounded their arguments in the empirical evidence, and expressed those arguments in clear and straightforward language, without scientific jargon. In doing so, they show that we know a good deal more about how our health system functions—and sometimes malfunctions—than the grandstanding and arguing around us suggest. As President Ronald Reagan once put it, "Facts are stubborn things." The facts about American health care should be at the center of the emerging debate over reform.

This volume grows out of a project hosted by the Social Science Research Council, "The Privatization of Risk." The goal of the project is to consider the extent to which the distribution, effect, and management of risks have changed over the last generation. Its particular subject is the *economic* risks facing Americans in the early twenty-first century: where they come from, whether and how they differ from those faced in the past, how people think about them, how governments and the private sector deal with them, and how they can better deal with them in the future.

This project is an effort to engage the social sciences constructively in important national policy discussions. Since the Progressive Era in the early twentieth century, social scientists have played a prominent role in the debate over economic security. Many of the early campaigners for public insurance programs (and some of their opponents) were themselves social scientists, or closely allied with the social sciences, especially the emerging economics profession. In calling for change, these social scientists believed they were bringing scientific principles to bear on pressing matters of public policy. In the years since, as economics, political science, sociology, and related disciplines have become more professional and specialized, social scientists have moved away from the front lines. But they have continued to contribute to economic policy discussions in numerous ways, studying the contours of America's distinctive welfare state, estimating the impact of specific government and private interventions, and developing proposals for change both targeted and sweeping.

The phrase "privatization of risk" traces two linked trends in the management of economic risk in the United States. The first is the contemporary celebration of the private sector as the first and best means of dealing with problems of all kinds. This enthusiasm for private-sector solutions is nothing new. Today, however, America's long-standing enthusiasm for the private sector is joined with a sometimes unbridled faith that new technologies and new attitudes have finally "solved" the problems of risk management that once bedeviled commercial insurers and private financial institutions. In this ascendant credo, not only should the private sector manage major risks; it can do it better than it ever has—and, needless to say, better than government ever could.

This brings us to the second trend: the shift of responsibility for managing economic risk from government and employers onto individuals and their families. I have elsewhere called this "the great risk shift," and I believe it is a defining economic (and political) transformation of our times.[2] The individual management of the economic risks of modern capitalism, whether through private retirement accounts or individual health savings accounts or through personal investments in education and housing, has never been as widespread or as widely celebrated as it is today. Yet with this responsibility has come pressing new questions about the ability of individuals to perceive, plan for, and secure themselves against the most threatening risks to their financial welfare—including the risks posed by declining health coverage and rising medical costs.

Each of the chapters that follow is concerned with one or more dimensions of the privatization of risk in American health care. How has health security changed in the United States? What is driving the change? What are its implications for the quality and cost of medical care received by Americans, or the health coverage they have (or, increasingly, do not have)? And what might be done to improve health security today? Although the authors are recognized experts, they have written their contributions so that they are accessible to interested nonexperts—which, ideally, should include a broad cross-section of Americans, so important is this discussion to us all.

The chapters in this volume do not present a single view on these questions. Nor are they of one mind about what should be done. What unites them is a commitment to grapple with three questions. First, what does social science research tell us about the interrelated problems that have prompted renewed attention to national health reform, most notably, those that are seen to compromise health security? Second, what does this research suggest with regard to how these problems should be addressed? Third, what does this research indicate about the prospects for changes of this sort? Not all of the contributors to this volume have addressed all three of these questions in depth, but each has thought about how his or her own research and the work of other social scientists illuminate the dimensions of contemporary problems as well as inform potential solutions to these problems.

Thus, in the first chapter, "The Transformation of American Health Insurance," Jill Quadagno and Brandon McKelvey, of the Pepper Institute on Aging and Public Policy at Florida State University, trace the changing ideology and institutions of American health insurance, looking at both the private and the public sectors. They focus on a revealing shift in how health insurance is understood to function: from an emphasis on shared risk, embodied in the traditional practice of "community rating," employed by public programs and some nonprofit insurers that did not charge higher rates to less healthy subscribers, toward an emphasis on individual risk management, embodied in the contemporary private practice of "experience rating," in which subscribers are charged according to their expected medical costs. The apotheosis of this shift, they suggest, are so-called Health Savings Accounts, tax-favored savings accounts that are coupled with a high-deductible "catastrophic" health plan, requiring that people pay most routine medical costs themselves. Although Quadagno and McKelvey are clearly worried about this new entrant into the insurance mix—they argue, based on strong evidence, that it is likely to fragment the market and drive up costs for many by encouraging healthier people to opt out of employment-based insurance—their broader point is that private health insurance is less and less a guarantee of the broad sharing of risk, leaving government and individuals to pick up the slack.

This point is driven home by Katherine Swartz in her chapter, "Uninsured in America: New Realties, New Risks." A Harvard economist, Swartz provides an informative tour of the uneven landscape of American health coverage. She tackles the big questions that should be at the heart of today's policy discussion: Who is most likely to be uninsured, and why? What are the key trends in coverage? And what are the options for creating broad risk-sharing in American health insurance given these trends? Swartz reminds us that the fundamental problems are relatively simple: Health insurance is too costly for middle- and working-class Americans, much less the poor, to finance reliably on their own. At the same time, because medical costs are so high, insurance is essential. The small share of Americans who end up incurring the lion's share of national health costs in any given year must have insurance to finance these expenditures. Yet insurance coverage is dwindling, and will likely to continue to dwindle as long as costs rise and employers see declining reason to offer coverage.

Not only the uninsured are at risk because of rising costs, remind Elizabeth Warren and Deborah Thorne in their chapter, "Get Sick, Go

Broke." So too are those who have coverage, either because they are "underinsured" or because they do not have protection for one big cost of sickness, time out of the workforce. Warren of Harvard Law School and Thorne of the Department of Sociology and Anthropology at Ohio University designed the pioneering Consumer Bankruptcy Project—a study that has used surveys, bankruptcy court records, interviews, and other evidence to look at rates and causes of bankruptcy filings over the past decade and a half. They have found that medical costs and crises are a leading (and probably increasing) cause of bankruptcy filings. Warren and Thorne discuss why medical bankruptcy is so common, affecting as many as 2.2 million Americans (filers and their dependents) in 2001; why it affects even those who have health insurance, who make up a surprising 75 percent of filers; and what can be done to reduce the problem.

Swartz, Warren, and Thorne are mainly interested in health security—whether people have insurance, whether they can afford care, and what happens when they do not or cannot. But the quality of medical care is also a crucial issue in American debates, with many critics of proposals to expand health security arguing that reform will hurt "the best medical care in the world." In the fourth chapter of this volume, I collaborate with noted health policy experts David Meltzer and Elizabeth A. McGlynn to bring recent research to bear on this topic, asking "Just How Good *Is* American Medical Care?" As a leading quality analyst for the RAND Corporation, McGlynn has led the charge in developing new measures that reveal how big the gap is between what is known to improve health and what is done by doctors and hospitals in the United States. The cornerstone of this research is a comprehensive database of clinical guidelines for the treatment of a range of acute and chronic health conditions—in essence, a yardstick against which the appropriateness of care delivered (or not delivered) to patients can be judged.

In this chapter we walk through the findings of this research: American adults receive only half of recommended care, children slightly less, and patients are more likely to be undertreated than overtreated. We then look at the United States in cross-national perspective, concluding that while American health care looks relatively good in comparative relief, it is hardly as exceptional as commonly believed. Despite the American system's very high price tag, for example, the United States has fewer doctors, hospital beds, and nurses per person than the norm among rich nations. Though less healthy overall than citizens of other rich nations, Americans visit doctors and hospitals less frequently and have shorter hospital stays. And the United States lags behind other rich nations in the use of information technology, such as electronic prescription systems, to improve quality and lower costs. Perhaps most surprising, the best care in the United States is actually delivered by the government: through the Veterans Health Administration, which, thanks in part to the innovative use of information technology, provides more than two-thirds of recommended care (vs. the 44–55 percent seen in the U.S. system overall). The big message is that quality does not naturally follow from greater spending or coverage; it needs to be cultivated with targeted efforts using information technology, practice guidelines, and other strategies for bringing into greater harmony what is known to work and what is actually done.

The cumulative effect of these chapters is to suggest that long-standing problems in American health care are growing worse even though there are known ways to make the situation better. The issue, it seems, is not irresolvable gaps in our knowledge or administrative capacities, but rather political and ideological disagreement about the proper direction of change. Given this evident dissensus, how likely is major action by our elected leaders to address declining health security? This is the question that I address in chapter 5, "The New Push for American Health Security." The goal of the chapter is to situate current political struggles in historical and cross-national relief. This requires knowing why the United States is the only affluent nation without health insurance for all its citizens, and what the answer to that question means for the prospects for reform today. It turns out that the main barrier to reform today is the failure of reform in the past, which has left the United States with a patchwork quilt of public and private coverage that divides the public and political elites and makes many Americans worried about the effect of change on *their* pieces of the quilt. In recent years, however, fundamental political and economic trends have collided to make large-scale reform a real possibility. The unanswered question is whether those favoring reform can learn from the "lessons of the past" and build a political and policy strategy that surmounts the barriers to reform that still loom large, without giving up on the basic aim of universal health security.

These contributions stand on their own. But they share a common conviction: that careful scholarship can and should speak to society directly and clearly on questions about which nonscholars truly care. The past and future of American health security could not be a more appropriate topic for such a discussion.

Every book rests on the contributions, advice, and assistance of many. That is all the more true of edited volumes. Each of the contributors to this book deserves a deep thanks. So too do the many colleagues, research assistants, administrative associates, spouses, friends, and children who directly or indirectly aided in the effort. Among them, Victoria Bilski deserves special gratitude for her diligent work transforming the essays that make up this volume into coherent and polished chapters.

Not only is this book inherently a collective effort, but in addition, it took a good deal of shared work to both envision it and bring it into its current printed form. All credit ultimately goes back to Craig Calhoun, president of the SSRC, who commissioned the "Privatization of Risk" project and envisioned the edited series that came out of it. Generous financial support for the project came from the John D. and Catherine T. MacArthur Foundation, as well as the SSRC itself.

To shepherd the volume to its completion, heartfelt thanks go to Paul Price at the SSRC and all of the hardworking editors and staff at Columbia University Press. They learned that it can be very difficult to contribute to current public debates, at least when that means turning a manuscript into a book in the amount of time that it takes most academic books to come back from reviewers. May the speed and quality of their efforts be a harbinger of the success of the debate that this book aims to influence.

NOTES

1   Previous debates took place during the 1930s, late 1940s, 1970s, and, of course, the early 1990s. I do not in this tally include the 1960s debate over Medicare, a program explicitly limited to the aged (though passed alongside the Medicaid program for the poor and later extended to the disabled). I say "at least the fifth" because there were arguably two major debates over reform in the 1970s—one

of which centered around President Nixon's proposal to mandate that employers provide coverage, the other of which occurred later in the decade and featured competing proposals by President Carter and Senator Kennedy, among others.

2   Jacob S. Hacker, *The Great Risk Shift: The New Economic Insecurity and the Decline of the American Dream*, rev. and exp. ed. (New York: Oxford University Press, 2008; originally published 2006).

CHAPTER ONE

The Transformation of American Health Insurance

JILL QUADAGNO & J. BRANDON MCKELVEY

Each year for more than a quarter century, the number of people without health insurance has continued to rise, to forty-seven million in 2007.[1] The only reason the situation does not look worse is that the government is picking up the slack—through Medicare and Medicaid and through the coverage provided to public employees. As public debate once again turns to the lack of health insurance, the choices offered differ in fundamental ways. At one end of the political spectrum are those who would base reform on a social insurance model, where risks are pooled broadly and costs distributed widely so that no individual or family has to fully bear the burden.[2] An alternative vision, which has become increasingly prominent since the mid-1990s, is consumer-directed health care (CDHC), a market-driven model based on the assumption that Americans should take greater responsibility for their own health care expenses.

CDHC advocates believe that the problem is not that people have too little insurance but that they have too much. They argue that excess insurance encourages wasteful consumption because it shields patients from the actual cost of care—the so-called moral hazard risk.[3] The goal of the CDHC movement is to transform patients into informed consumers by making medical care a commodity that is purchased in the same way as other market goods.[4] Presumably, if individuals are forced to pay a larger share of their health care expenses, they will shop more carefully and "purchase" only those services that they really need or are of proven value.[5] As demand for unnecessary medical services declines, costs will go down, making coverage more affordable for everyone.

The goal of CDHC, to increase cost sharing and promote cost awareness, is being met through health savings accounts (HSAs) coupled with high deductible plans for "catastrophic" expenses, in a radical shift from defined-benefit to defined-contribution employer plans and through an expanded role for private insurance companies in the public programs, Medicaid and Medicare. This transition has been implemented through obscure changes in tax law, technocratic provisions added to bills designed for other purposes, experiments with Medicaid "waivers," and a new option, Medicare Advantage. Taken together these policy changes have begun to transform health care financing in both the public and private arena.

CDHC is fundamentally at odds with the social insurance principle, which provides a guarantee of protection, regardless of income or health status. Over the long run, it could undermine the comprehensive private benefits that offered near universal coverage within the workplace and the public social insurance programs that have protected the aged, disabled, and poor. How did CDHC become a viable political option when just forty years ago the goal of universal social insurance seemed imminent? And what are the implications for quality, cost, and coverage?

THE UNREALIZED PROMISE OF UNIVERSAL COVERAGE

The foundation of the current health care system was constructed in the post–World War II era when, in the wake of President Harry Truman's failed proposal for national health insurance, the trade unions embarked on a campaign to negotiate health benefits in their collective bargaining agreements. As unions won comprehensive health benefits for workers and their dependents, nonunionized firms followed suit. By the late 1950s more than half of all Americans had health insurance through their jobs. The enactment of Medicare and Medicaid in 1965 extended health coverage to the elderly and provided a safety net for the poor.

Although social reformers were convinced that national health insurance was the inevitable next step, the dream was never realized.

Medicare had solved the problem of insuring the aged, but it also fueled inflation, causing health care costs to rise significantly.[6] Inflation, coupled with a souring economy in the 1970s, reduced prospects for expanding government obligations, a situation that lent credence to conservatives' view that the welfare state was a drain on the economy.

Rising health care costs not only affected Medicare spending but spilled over to private payers as well. As employers' expenditures for health benefits grew, by 700 percent between 1970 and 1982, they began seeking ways to escape from the commitments they had made to fully pay employees' medical expenses.[7] At first managed care appeared to offer a way to contain inflation in medical expenditures. Between 1984 and 1999, health maintenance organizations (HMOs) and other managed care arrangements increased their share of the private benefits market from 7 to 85 percent.[8] Although managed care did produce short-term savings, it failed to live up to its promises over the long term. Moreover, the HMOs' aggressive cost containment measures angered physicians who objected to restraints on their professional autonomy and patients who resented what they perceived as unjust rationing of medical services. In the 1990s patients joined with physicians in a consumer revolt against some of the more egregious managed care practices, resulting in federal mandates on hospital stays for childbirth and mastectomies and numerous restrictions in the states.[9]

Once again medical costs resumed their upward spiral, forcing employers to seek new ways to reduce their health care obligations. Between 2000 and 2005, the percent of businesses offering health benefits declined from 69 to 60 percent, with most of the erosion occurring among small firms. By 2005 only 47 percent of the smallest of firms, those with three to nine employees, offered health benefits.[10] Employers also shed their long-term obligations to retirees, with the percent of large firms that paid retiree health benefits dropping from 66 percent in 1988 to 33 percent by 2007.[11]

THE ORIGINS OF HEALTH SAVINGS ACCOUNTS

The current panacea for controlling costs has come in the form of the HSA, a kind of medical IRA. This idea was first promoted by John Goodman, the president of a corporate-funded think tank, the National Center for Policy Analysis (NCPA), and Richard Rahn, chief economist of the Chamber of Commerce of the United States, as a way to phase out Medicare.[12] In a 1984 *Wall Street Journal* article, Goodman and Rahn argued for privatizing Medicare by allowing individuals to make deposits into medical savings accounts (MSAs) during their working years and then draw upon these funds to pay for private health insurance in retirement. Over the long term, Medicare would be replaced by private coverage.

Although the Medicare reform plan gained no supporters at the time, Goodman began a campaign to promote MSAs in private health plans. One of the first companies to experiment with them was Golden Rule Insurance Company, a firm known for aggressive underwriting policies and battles with regulators over insurance reform in the states.[13] In 1994 Golden Rule added to its product line MSAs coupled with a no-frills health insurance policy. MSAs failed to spread, however, because funds contributed to them had no tax advantage over other types of plans.[14] What was needed was a political campaign to convince Congress to support legislation that would create a more favorable tax situation.[15]

To win favor for MSAs in Congress, Golden Rule became one of the single largest donors to political campaigns, contributing $1,069,000 in 1993–94, mostly to Republicans. An important ally was the Council for Affordable Health Insurance (CAHI), an organization of the smaller insurers that had lost market share due to the trend toward managed care that favored the large HMOs and to a more general erosion of the commercial insurance industry. The erosion began following enactment of the Employer Retirement Income Security Act (ERISA) of 1973. ERISA excluded self-insured plans from state regulations mandating that health plans include specific benefits and exempted them from federal and state taxes.[16] Following ERISA the majority of large employers became self-insured. Rather than paying premiums to insurers, they withdrew their health benefit dollars from insurance premium pools and put them in benefit trusts. Self-funding allowed companies to keep the interest on the funds in the trusts, better time payments to meet their cash flow cycles, and avoid state taxes on premiums. It also liberated them from mandated benefits that commercial insurance plans had to include. As self-insured firms cut their overhead costs, insurance companies were pushed into the less lucrative business of claims processing, reinsuring these firms against large losses, and/or selling to small businesses that lacked the resources and administrative capacity to self-insure. The result was an erosion of the economic base of commercial insurance plans. Between 1965 and 1985 the market share of commercial insurance companies declined from 55 to 35 percent. Insurers also lost a major revenue source through loss of interest on deposits.[17] MSAs provided an opportunity to introduce a new product into their shrunken market.[18]

In the 1994 congressional elections, Republicans controlled both the House and the Senate, and Rep. Newt Gingrich (R-GA) ascended to the position of Speaker of the House. Over the next two years Golden Rule became one of Gingrich's largest donors. In 1995 the company contributed $25,000 to GOPAC, Gingrich's political action committee, $43,510 to Friends of Gingrich, his campaign committee, and $20,000 to the Progress and Freedom Foundation, a Washington think tank that sponsored Gingrich's Progress Report, which was broadcast on National Empowerment Television.[19] In return Gingrich promoted Golden Rule in his televised college course, praised MSAs in his book, *To Renew America,* and declared that MSAs were "the most exciting option we are going to offer."[20] Rep. Bill Archer (R-TX), a leading CDHC advocate, promised that MSAs would expand "freedom, choice, personal responsibility and savings."[21] NCPA president John Goodman agreed: "What medical savings accounts do is it gives people a little bit of freedom and a little bit of control over their own health care dollars so that every decision is not made by the managed care bureaucracy."[22]

The Health Insurance Portability and Accountability Act of 1996 (HIPAA) instituted several reforms designed to protect high-risk people against insurance underwriting practices. It gave employees who lost group coverage the right to convert those policies to individual coverage, prohibited insurers from charging different premiums for individuals within groups, and required insurers to guarantee renewal to any group. In exchange for their support, Republicans insisted on including tax subsidies to MSAs for the self-employed and small businesses on an experimental basis.[23] MSAs were given another boost when a pilot program for Medicare beneficiaries was tacked onto the Balanced Budget Act of 1997. Neither of these seemingly innocuous experiments suggested that MSAs had any future. Not a single beneficiary initially signed up for Medicare MSAs and so few people signed up for the HIPAA MSAs that the General Accounting Office was unable to evaluate their effects.[24]

The turning point for the CDHC movement came with the Medicare Modernization Act of 2003, which provided a prescription drug benefit and incentives for beneficiaries to switch from traditional Medicare to private managed care plans. What received virtually no attention at that time in the heated debates over the drug benefit was a provision that allowed an employee to establish a health savings account, as MSAs were now called. Employers or employees were allowed to contribute funds to an HSA up to the amount of the deductible, originally limited to $2,250 for an individual and $4,500 for a family. These accounts had to be coupled with a high deductible health insurance plan (HDHP) to pay for "catastrophic" care.[25]

Over the next two years, President Bush pushed to expand HSAs, explaining in a 2005 speech that "health savings accounts all aim at empowering people to make decisions for themselves, owning their own health care plan, and at the same time bringing some demand control into the cost of heath care."[26] In the waning hours of the 2006 Republican-controlled legislature, Congress enacted the Tax Relief and Health Care Act, which raised allowable HSA contributions, gave employees the right to roll over funds from other types of employer health spending accounts into HSAs, and permitted a one-time transfer of funds from IRAs into HSAs.[27] Thus, one of the unrecognized achievements of the Bush administration was to set in place policies that would move the health care system toward a consumer-directed vision with its emphasis on individuals' responsibility and away from the broad risk pooling protection afforded by social insurance.

HEALTH SAVINGS ACCOUNTS UNDER CURRENT LAW

CDHC plans operate differently from conventional insurance. Individuals are expected to use funds in the HSA to pay for basic medical expenses, including doctor's visits, prescription drugs, and elective surgery, or even items not usually covered by insurance such as premiums for long-term care insurance, nonprescription drugs, and lodging away from home for medical care. Individuals can also use the HSAs to pay for nonmedical expenses but have to pay a 10 percent tax penalty on the amount withdrawn. If an individual dies, becomes disabled, or reaches sixty-five, there are no limits on how accumulated funds can be spent.[28] Unlike other employer health spending accounts, unused funds in HSAs roll over from year to year and follow employees who change jobs.[29]

What is most revolutionary about HSAs is their treatment by the tax code. In no other arrangement are contributions, earnings, and withdrawals not subject to taxes. Contributions to HSAs can be made with pretax dollars. Earnings on HSA funds are allowed to accumulate on a tax-free basis. Withdrawals also are exempt from taxes as long as they are used to pay medical expenses.[30] Funds held in HSA accounts can be invested in various vehicles such as stocks and bonds, mutual funds, and even hedge funds, if the balance is large enough. Since there are no income limits on who is allowed to contribute, HSAs provide a lucrative new tax shelter for wealthier people. These plans are not as attractive to less affluent people, however, even though premiums may be lower, because out-of-pocket expenses are often higher.[31] Individuals who have HSA/HDHC plans can do well as long as they stay healthy. Should they become ill, however, their medical costs can substantially exceed their HSA savings.[32] In 2007 an employee with family coverage could pay as much as $11,200 in out-of-pocket medical costs before the catastrophic plan began to pay. Further, there is nothing in the law that prevents insurance companies from engaging in the pernicious forms of medical underwriting they currently use to cherry-pick customers.[33]

The larger threat posed by CDHC-type plans is to comprehensive employer benefit plans. If healthy, more affluent workers opt out of these comprehensive health plans in favor of HSA-type benefits, as is already happening, older and sicker people will be left in the pool. As a result, their premiums will rise significantly.[34] Rather than promoting personal responsibility, HSA/HDHC plans segment consumers into ever-smaller risk pools, making other types of coverage too expensive for most people. Those who benefit will be the insurers who sell in the small group market and employers who will use CDHC plans to shift costs to employees.

HSAs first became available in January 2004. Relatively few people currently have HSA/HDHC policies, because employees remain wary of assuming unpredictable risks. When offered a choice, only 19 percent of employees selected a CDHC plan.[35] However, these plans have spread among people who purchase insurance in the individual market. Most of the five thousand insurance plans from one hundred fifty different companies offered by eHealthInsurance.com, a website that helps individuals find affordable coverage, include HSA/HDHC plans. Employers have also begun to offer employees an HSA option in their benefit packages, believing these plans will help reduce costs.[36] Between 2005 and 2006 the percent of employers offering these plans increased from 2 to 6 percent.[37] Although HSAs were originally conceived as a product for individuals and small employers, nearly half of the 4.5 million people covered by HSAs in 2007 worked for firms with more than fifty employees.[38] In fact, the fastest growth is in the large group market.[39] In 2007 Mintel, a marketing research firm, predicted that the number of HSA enrollees would rise to thirty million by 2009.[40]

It is still unclear whether these optimistic predictions will materialize. One obstacle to CDHC is the political clout of the large HMOs. The Group Health Association of America, the organization that represents HMOs, warns that HSA/HDHC plans create "adverse selection against HMOs, because healthy individuals would opt for catastrophic coverage, leaving a high proportion of high-risk individuals in HMOs." The result would be an increase in premiums "for those remaining in comprehensive coverage arrangements."[41] Over the long run, MSAs could "reverse advances in the current marketplace by providing a tax advantage to old-style, uncoordinated, and inefficient health care coverage."[42]

State mandates requiring insurance companies to cover certain procedures and services pose another obstacle to the expansion of HSA/HDHC plans. Because mandates make it difficult for insurers to offer plans that only cover "catastrophic" costs, they have emerged as a key target in the battle over health care reform. Critics argue that these mandates are not based on rational scientific knowledge about best practices but rather cater to special interests that exert political pressure to force insurers to cover unnecessary or frivolous procedures and treatments, needlessly inflating the cost of health care. Although it is true that some mandates have been added to state regulations because of lobbying efforts, mandates also protect patients by forcing insurance plans to include a minimum level of basic services, such as immunizations for children. Eliminating them will force individuals to engage in complex forms of risk assessment, as they weigh their income constraints against their analysis of future health risk.[43]

CDHC advocates view comprehensive employer benefit plans as the primary source of inflation in medical costs. To reduce the "moral hazard" inherent in these plans, they advocate a switch from defined benefit (DB) plans to a defined contribution (DC) system. DC plans represent another way to shift risk from employers to individuals, a transition that has already occurred in pensions.

Until the late 1970s employer pension plans took the form of a defined benefit that guaranteed retired workers a fixed annuity with the amount determined by prior wages and years of service. In 1978 an obscure provision, section 401K, was added to the tax code allowing workers and employers to make contributions that would not be taxed until the worker retired. These defined contributions liberated employers from long-term obligations by making pension benefits a fixed payment.[44] In subsequent years, 401KS and their sister funds, Individual Retirement Accounts, expanded rapidly while traditional pensions declined. In the 1970s three-quarters of workers with pension coverage had a DB plan; by 2001 that figure had declined to 33 percent.[45]

DC health benefits are similar in concept to DC pensions. Employers contribute a set amount and employees then select the coverage they can afford based on their estimate of health risk. Instead of an open-ended entitlement embodied in most employer plans and in Medicare and Medicaid, DC plans cap third-party obligations and shift the risk of unexpected medical expenses to the individual.

It is possible that DC health benefits will follow the path of DC pension programs. A survey conducted in 1999 found that many employers were considering making the switch. According to a report by the consulting firm of Booz-Allen, nearly all of *Fortune* magazine's "100 Best Companies to Work For" were anticipating a shift to DC health plans and expected to save millions of dollars in administrative costs as a result. The report concluded that the move to DC health plans was three to five years away and that within ten years the DC system would become as common in health care as it is in retirement benefits.[46]

That transition has yet to materialize for several reasons. DC health benefits may be less expensive for employers and more compatible with a labor market where the concept of lifetime employment has eroded and where employees can expect to change jobs numerous times before they retire. The defined contribution concept works quite differently in health care, however, than it does in pensions. Whereas retirement savings fund future income expenditures, health insurance pays for current needs. Because the costs to individuals are immediately apparent, the transition will be more difficult to make. Further, private pensions, in whatever form, supplement the guaranteed income stream that Social Security provides. DC pensions have succeeded, in part, because Social Security provides a basic layer of protection against income loss due to retirement. There is no equivalent to Social Security in health care for people under age sixty-five.

CONSUMER-DIRECTED HEALTH CARE IN MEDICAID

Over the past decade, state Medicaid expenditures have been growing rapidly, squeezing out funds for other social needs. By 2006 Medicaid constituted 16 percent of state budgets on average. As a result, governors of both parties have been searching for ways to contain Medicaid growth. The problem is that while states have some discretionary power to determine benefits, they are also constrained by numerous federal regulations about what groups must be covered and what services must be provided. Further, Medicaid is an entitlement, which means that the federal government matches state spending for services on an open-ended basis with no upper limit. This formula creates a dilemma. On the one hand, states have incentives to expand Medicaid enrollment because it brings increased federal dollars. On the other hand, Medicaid costs automatically increase as states contribute their share of the matching funds for each qualified beneficiary.[47]

In 2000 the National Governors Association formed a bipartisan task force to develop a plan for reducing Medicaid expenditures. Although the governors on the task force agreed on the necessity of greater flexibility to tailor program needs to different population groups, Republicans also requested federal permission to "design benefit packages to look more like commercial models," to "promote personal responsibility," to "make Medicaid beneficiaries share the cost of their care," and to "encourage choice through private health insurance." The biggest impediment to a bipartisan agreement, however, was a Republican demand that the federal government change Medicaid from an open-ended entitlement "without responsibility" to a block grant within a fixed budget.[48] Block granting would mean that states would be freed from some federal regulations about what groups must be covered and what services must be provided. It would end Medicaid's status as an entitlement.[49]

Some of the Republican proposals for Medicaid reform were incorporated into the Deficit Reduction Act of 2005, which allowed states to impose cost sharing on Medicaid beneficiaries and authorized ten state demonstrations of Health Opportunity Accounts (HOAs).[50] The intent of the HOAs is to reduce moral hazard by giving states a mechanism to monitor beneficiaries so as to prevent them from faking their medical problems or engaging in behaviors that increase their exposure to risk.

States are testing two models under the options available, either alone or in some combination. The first is the direct services model, in which the state funds an HOA for each Medicaid beneficiary to encourage healthy behaviors. Beneficiaries can use their HOA funds to pay for deductibles, co-payments, and extra health expenses. If they lose their Medicaid eligibility through employment, they can use their HOA funds to buy into an employer's health plan. States are also testing an insurance model in which each Medicaid beneficiary receives a premium payment, essentially a voucher, to apply toward a state-approved insurance plan.[51] The larger objective of these experiments is to make Medicaid more like DC benefits in the private health insurance market. Instead of purchasing health care services, the states' task will be to facilitate a Medicaid marketplace.[52]

As states have restructured their Medicaid programs, they have adopted language and policies that reflect the rhetoric of consumer-directed health care. Florida's HMO Advantage will create "a new Medicaid program that recognizes the individual's role in planning and purchasing health services."[53] Its ultimate objective is to fundamentally transform relationships, responsibilities, and economic incentives and allow market competition to "inspire innovation and efficiency."[54] Similarly, when Massachusetts Governor Mitt Romney signed into law the Massachusetts Health Care Reform Plan in 2006, he touted his plan as a way to provide nearly universal coverage to state residents through "a single consumer-driven marketplace for health insurance for small businesses, their employees and individuals."[55]

The Massachusetts plan includes a mandate that requires employers with eleven or more employees to make a "fair and reasonable" contribution toward their employees' health benefits or pay an annual fee.[56] It also contains an individual mandate requiring all residents eighteen and over to purchase health insurance. To shore up the individual/small group insurance market, Massachusetts created the Commonwealth Health Insurance Connector. Firms that designate the Connector as their employer-sponsored plan will be allowed to make contributions to pay for employee health benefits on a pretax basis. To reduce the cost of coverage, plans sold through the Connector will be exempt from some state mandates. Mandate-free insurance will be offered to young adults aged nineteen to twenty-six at a reduced cost.[57] Younger people are likely to prefer the HSA/high deductible option, because these plans will have low premiums. As they gain experience with this type of plan and build savings in HSA accounts, they will likely become a political pressure group to extend mandate-free coverage to other age groups. Thus, through a combination of incentives and subsidies, the Massachusetts plan reinforces the individual and small group insurance market in a way that will promote the growth of the HSA market.[58]

CONSUMER-DIRECTED HEALTH CARE IN MEDICARE

Medicare, the federal program of health insurance for the elderly and disabled, is facing many of the same troubles as Medicaid. The problem of rising health care costs is exacerbated by the aging of the population. According to the Medicare trustees, by 2018 the trust fund will have a shortfall, requiring large transfers from income tax revenues to cover the expected deficit.[59] As Congress tackles Medicare reform, the pressing issue is whether the program will be preserved as an entitlement or whether even the elderly and disabled will be subject to the dictates of consumer-directed care.

When Republicans gained control of Congress in 1994, they sought to implement provisions that would allow Medicare to eventually self-destruct. As Gingrich explained in a speech to hospitals officials: Medicare was like "Soviet-style health care—too bureaucratic, too centralized and too dominated by government."[60] He would scrap existing Medicare rules, which limited sales of private insurance to supplemental

"Medigap" policies, and give beneficiaries the option of withdrawing from Medicare and using their share of funds to purchase private coverage. Thus, the main goal was to open the entire Medicare beneficiary market to private insurers.[61]

In the past few years, Congress has enacted measures that have given private insurers a larger role in Medicare, most recently with the Medicare Modernization Act of 2003, which created Medicare Advantage, a private insurance option. There is already evidence that inserting private insurance into a social insurance program exposes beneficiaries to the risk of abuse. The private insurers that run Medicare's new drug benefit program and offer other private insurance options encouraged by the Bush administration have used deceptive sales tactics and improperly denied claims to thousands of beneficiaries. The problems include improper termination of coverage for people with HIV and AIDS, huge backlogs of claims and complaints, and a failure to answer telephone calls. In 2007 Medicare imposed more than $770,000 in fines on eleven companies for marketing violations and for failing to notify beneficiaries about changes in costs and benefits in a timely fashion.[62] Many of the marketing abuses occurred in sales of the Medicare Advantage product.

Another option favored by CDHC advocates is to allow younger workers to deposit some or all of their Medicare payroll taxes into a personal HSA account for their future health care needs. When they reach retirement age, they would use these funds to purchase private coverage. Over the long term, Medicare would become a privately financed program.[63]

The larger goal of the CDHC movement is to fully convert Medicare into a DC system. Under a DC system each beneficiary would receive a voucher, which could be supplemented with private funds, to purchase private health insurance and/or to deposit into an HSA. Converting Medicare into a DC system would create multiple insurance pools, undermining the program's redistributive aspects and reducing its risk-spreading features. As has happened with private insurance, insurers could use subtle tactics to recruit younger, healthier seniors, leaving the oldest, sickest beneficiaries in the traditional program. Premiums, deductibles, and co-payments would inevitably have to rise for this vulnerable population.[64] Further, the money sitting in HSA accounts would no longer be available to Medicare, forcing the government to increase spending or decrease care, creating a death spiral. But that is the plan. According to

Gingrich: "We don't want to get rid of it in round one because we don't think it's politically smart. But we believe that it's going to wither on the vine because we think [seniors] are going to leave it voluntarily."[65]

THE LIMITS OF CONSUMER-DIRECTED HEALTH CARE

In the nearly half century since Medicare was enacted, cost containment efforts have primarily been directed toward controlling the behavior of providers. Consumer-directed health care is based on a different premise, that of changing the behavior of the patient. It revolves around the logic of moral hazard, that people overconsume health care because insurance buffers them from the actual cost of medical services. Its proposed solution is to make patients more cost conscious.

People do consume less health care when they pay a portion of the costs.[66] The problem is that most patients have no way of knowing in advance which care is useful and which is wasteful and often reduce useful care and unnecessary care equally.[67] A major worry is that low-income people, in particular, will skimp on preventive care to "save" their funds for future unknowable expenses. In the long run, costs would be higher because people who forgo prevention have illnesses diagnosed at later stages when they are more difficult to treat. A Kaiser Family Foundation survey suggests that this is already happening.[68] Compared to people in traditional plans, enrollees in HSA/HDHC plans are less likely to fill a prescription, more likely to skip a recommended test, and more likely to say they went without medical care.

Consumer-directed health care also presumes an unproven causal relationship between individual consumption decisions and the costs of health care. A large proportion of the recent rise in health care spending is due to an increase in the treatment of diseases that in the past might have gone untreated. It is also due to innovations in medical care, causes over which patients have little control.[69] Other factors that affect the growth in health spending, such as greater use of prescription drugs, higher enrollment in Medicaid, technological innovations, and care of the chronically ill, are unlikely to be responsive to consumer-directed solutions.[70] Further, CDHC plans do cover large health care expenditures, and it is these expenses that drive health care costs, not the relatively minor out-of-pocket expenses.

Other nations that have adopted a CDHC approach provide lessons about the possible consequences for the United States. In South Africa about half of privately insured individuals have MSA/high deductible plans. These plans have become a tool for insurance companies to attract the young and healthy, leaving older, sicker people in non-MSA type plans.[71] Singapore also instituted an HSA-type program called Medisave in 1994. Although Medisave appears to have successfully controlled costs, it differs in significant ways from the model favored by CDHC advocates in the United States.[72] Medisave is one component of a countrywide *compulsory* savings program. Employers and employees are required to contribute 40 percent of gross salary to their Medisave accounts, which also can be used for retirement and other large expenditures. The mandatory savings provision alone would likely preclude such a plan from being adopted in the United States. More importantly, in Singapore, the government is the main health care provider. The government not only sets the amount Medisave funds pay for hospital care and physician services but also limits expenditures to necessary medical care and excludes nonessential procedures.[73] The illusion that health care costs are low because of cautious consumer spending actually reflects strict government rationing of services. Further, only 7.7 percent of Singapore's population is sixty-five or older, compared to nearly 13 percent in the United States. Thus, in regard to ideology, characteristics of the health care system, and demographics, Singapore is a poor model for the United States to emulate.

For decades the employment-based health insurance system that was constructed in the 1940s has been unraveling at the seams. Continually rising health care costs have reduced employer commitment to health benefits and opened the market to new forms of coverage. Until the mid-1990s, it appeared that managed care would trump fee-for-service as the predominant method of financing and delivering health care services. Although managed care has its flaws, it does not stray from and indeed reinforces the concepts of shared risk, comprehensive benefits, and preventive care that characterize the employer benefit system.

The trend toward managed care placed the mid-sized insurers that operated in the individual and small group market at a competitive disadvantage with the large HMOs, and they seized upon CDHC as a way to increase their market share. In the past five years, the Bush administration has engineered changes in the tax code that have helped improve the market position of these companies. A consumer-driven health care revolution has begun, and the key question is whether it will shape the direction the health care system will take in the future.

On the one hand, CDHC has become the preferred solution of many who are involved in the vast network of interest groups and constituencies that have been constructed around the existing health care system over the past seventy years and who have successfully opposed previous efforts at health care reform.[74] The major insurers already offer an HSA option and the Health Insurance Association of America has been lobbying Congress to eliminate the obstacles to expansion.[75] The American Medical Association also favors a defined contribution system, tax credits, and HSA/HDHC plans.[76] Employers are attracted to HSA/HDHC plans because they reduce their administrative costs and make their health expenditures more predictable. Even some Democrats, particularly those who represent rural areas, favor HSA/HDHC plans because managed care functions poorly in these regions. Financial institutions, too, have found administering HSAs to be highly lucrative. Although the main objective for banks is to increase deposit income, HSA management also generates income from fees for account processing. Interestingly, some insurance companies, like Blue Cross, have started handling their own banking services, blurring the boundary between banks and insurance.[77] These new allies have become part of the pressure group to eliminate disincentives to HSAs in federal law.

On the other hand, the trade unions are ambivalent, the large HMOs are opposed, and the public remains wary. Further, although the Republican Party has chosen a consumer-directed model as the solution to the problems plaguing the health care system, this may not be a politically viable choice. Even though younger and higher income employees may prefer these plans because of the tax advantages and lower premiums, people who hold consumer-directed plans rate their insurance lower on overall performance, are less satisfied with what they pay, would be more likely to change coverage in the future, and feel more vulnerable to health care costs.[78] Moreover, it is the target population of CDHC — wealthier, better-educated, healthier people — who are most likely to have these reservations. It is unclear whether the unprecedented tax advantages of HSAs are sufficient to overcome these concerns in the long run. Because the incentives for CDHC have been constructed without the public debate that usually accompanies major policy initiatives, policymakers have thus far not been held accountable.

Although there have been numerous attempts over the past quarter century to downsize the welfare state by tinkering with benefit formulas and reimbursement systems, these changes did not alter the core structure of health benefits. The CDHC movement represents a more fundamental restructuring that transforms the underlying principles of both direct public health benefits and private publicly subsidized benefits. The shift toward consumer-directed health care could signify the final phase in the erosion of the comprehensive employer benefit plans that approached a social insurance model in the workplace and a radical shift in the underlying constructs of the public programs that have protected the elderly, the disabled, and the poor against the risk of being unable to afford coverage or being rejected because they are sick.

NOTES

Acknowledgment: We thank Timothy Stoltzfus Jost and Jacob S. Hacker for helpful comments on a previous draft of this chapter.

1   U.S. Census Bureau, *Current Population Survey* (2007), http://www.census.gov/Press-Release/www/releases/archives/income_wealth/010583.html.

2   Jacob S. Hacker, *The Great Risk Shift: The New Economic Insecurity and the Decline of the American Dream,* rev. and exp. ed. (New York: Oxford University Press, 2008; originally published 2006).

3   Mark Pauly, "The Economics of Moral Hazard," *American Economic Review* 58 (1968): 531–37.

4   Pauly, "Economics of Moral Hazard"; Malcolm Gladwell, "The Moral-Hazard Myth: The Bad Idea Behind Our Failed Health Care System," *The New Yorker,* August 8, 2005, 1–10.

5   Pauly, "Economics of Moral Hazard"; John Nyman, *The Theory of the Demand for Health Insurance* (Palo Alto: Stanford University Press, 2003).

6   Jill Quadagno, *One Nation, Uninsured: Why the U.S. Has No National Health Insurance* (New York: Oxford University Press, 2005); Theodore Marmor, *The Politics of Medicare,* 2nd ed. (New York: Aldine de Gruyter, 2000).

7   Linda Bergthold, *Purchasing Power in Health* (New Brunswick: Rutgers University Press, 1990).

8   Greg Scandlen, "Defined Contribution Health Insurance," *Policy Backgrounder No. 154*, National Center for Policy Analysis, October 26, 2000, http://www.ncpa.org/bg/bg154/bg154html.

9   Quadagno, *One Nation, Uninsured*.

10 Kaiser Family Foundation, *Employer Health Benefits: 2006 Survey of Findings* (Menlo Park, CA: Henry J. Kaiser Family Foundation, 2006), http://www.kff.org/insurance/7527/upload/7528.pdf.

11 Jyoti Thottam, "GM's Get-Well Plan," *Time*, October 1, 2007, 53–54.

12 John Goodman and Richard Rahn, "Salvaging Medicare with an IRA," *Wall Street Journal*, March 20, 1984, 1.

13 Charles R. Rateliff, Testimony of Charles R. Rateliff, Senior Vice President, Benefits Administration and Risk Management, Wal-Mart Stores, Inc. before the Subcommittee on Health, Committee on Ways and Means, House of Representatives, June 27, 1995, pp. 80–81.

14 Michael Cannon, "Health Savings Accounts: Do the Critics Have a Point?" *Cato Institute Policy Analysis No. 569*, May 30, 2006, http://www.cato.org/pub_display.php?pub_id=6395.

15 John Goodman, *Patient Power: The Free Market Alternative to Clinton's Health Plan* (Washington, DC: The Cato Institute, 1993).

16 Timothy S. Jost and Mark Hall, "The Role of State Regulation in Consumer-Driven Health Care," *American Journal of Law and Medicine* 31 (2005): 395–418.

17 Jeff Goldsmith, "Death of a Paradigm: The Challenge of Competition," *Health Affairs* 3, no. 3 (1990): 5–19.

18 William Bowen, "Policy Innovation and Health Insurance Reform in the American States: An Event History Analysis of State Medical Savings Account Adoptions (1993–1996)" (PhD diss., Florida State University, 2003).

19 Robert Dreyfuss and Peter H. Stone, "Medikill: Golden Rule Insurance has lavished campaign funds on Gingrich and the GOP in order to promote its medical savings account scheme—and destroy Medicare," *Mother Jones* (January/February 1996): 1–8.

20 Common Cause, "Politically Insured, Doctor Recommended: Health Insurance and Doctors Give Nearly $50 million in Pac and Soft Money Contributions During Last Decade." *Common Cause News*, December 1, 1995, 5. http://www.ccsi.com/~comcause/news/medical.html.

21 Ibid., 26.

22 Ibid., 65.

23 Hacker, *The Great Risk Shift*.

24 Timothy S. Jost, "Our Broken Health Care System and How to Fix It; An Essay on Health Law and Policy," *Wake Forest Law Review* 41 (2006): 537–618; Timothy S. Jost, *Health Care at Risk: A Critique of the Consumer-Driven Movement* (Durham, NC: Duke University Press, 2007).

25 Hacker, *The Great Risk Shift*.

26 Michael Fletcher, "Bush Promotes Health Savings Accounts," *Washington Post*, January 27, 2005, A2.

27 U.S. Department of Treasury, "Health Savings Accounts HSAs," 2006, http://www.ustreas.gov/.

28 Jost, "Our Broken Health Care System."

29 Cannon, "Health Savings Accounts."

30 Edwin Park and Robert Greenstein, "Latest Enrollment Data Still Fail to Dispel Concerns about Health Savings Accounts," Center on Budget and Policy Priorities, January 30, 2006, http://www.chpp.org/10-26-05health2.htm.

31 Jon Gabel, Jeremy Pickreign, and Heidi Whitmore, "Behind the Slow Growth of Employer-Based Consumer-Directed Health Plans," Center for Studying Health System Change, *Issue Brief No. 107*, December 2006, http://www.hschange.com/CONTENT/900/.

32 Hacker, *The Great Risk Shift*.

33 Donald Light, "The Practice and Ethics of Risk-Related Health Insurance," *JAMA* 267 (1992): 2503–04.

34 Marilyn Moon, Len Nichols, and Susan Wall, *Medical Savings Accounts: A Policy Analysis* (Washington, DC: Urban Institute, 1996), http://www.urban.org/msa.pdf.

35 Kaiser Family Foundation, *Employer Health Benefits*.

36 Cannon, "Health Savings Accounts."

37 Kaiser Family Foundation, *National Survey of Enrollees in Consumer-Directed Health Plans* (Menlo Park, CA: Kaiser Family Foundation, November 2006).

38 Jerry Geisel, "HSA Contribution Limits Set to Increase," *AIG Passport*, posted May 14, 2007, 12:43 PM, http://www.businessinsurance.com/cgi-bin/news,pl?newsId=10203.

39 Joanne Wojcik, "Large Employers Lead in HSA Adoption," Podcast, posted April 2, 2007, 2:52 PM, http://www.businessinsurance.com/cgi-bin/news,pl?newsId=9899.

40 Mintel, "Mintel Report Predicts Health Savings Account Enrollees to Rise to 30

Million by 2009," May 22, 2007, http://www.health--savings--accounts.com/hsa-weblog-arch/2007/05/mintel_report_p.html.

41 Group Health Association of America, Statement of the Group Health Association of America for the Subcommittee on Health, Committee on Ways and Means, House of Representatives, June 27, 1995, 112.

42 Ibid.,114.

43 Nyman, *The Theory of the Demand for Health Insurance.*

44 Scandlen, "Defined Contribution Health Insurance."

45 William Even and David Macpherson, "Defined Contribution Plans and the Distribution of Pension Wealth," *Industrial Relations* 46, no. 3 (2007): 551–58.

46 Scandlen, "Defined Contribution Health Insurance."

47 Vernon Smith, Rekha Ramesh, Kathleen Gifford, Eileen Ellis, Robin Rudowitz, and Molly O'Malley, *The Continuing Medicaid Budget Challenge: State Medicaid Spending Growth and Cost Containment in Fiscal Years 2005 and 2005,* Kaiser Commission on Medicaid and the Uninsured (Menlo Park, CA: Henry J. Kaiser Family Foundation, October, 2004).

48 Letter from Republican Governors Jeb Bush (FL), John Rowland (CT), and Bill Owens (CO) to President George Bush and HHS Secretary Tommy Thompson, January 16, 2003; files of Dr. Lori Parham, State Director, AARP Florida.

49 Smith et al., "The Continuing Medicaid Budget Challenge."

50 Charles Milligan, Cynthia Woodcock, and Alice Burton, "Turning Medicaid Beneficiaries into Purchasers of Health Care: Critical Success Factors of Medicaid Consumer-Directed Health Purchasing," Academy Health, Robert Wood Johnson Foundation, *State Coverage Initiatives* (January 2006); Kaiser Commission on Medicaid and the Uninsured, *Low Medicaid Spending Growth Amid Rebounding State Revenues* (Menlo Park, CA: Henry J. Kaiser Family Foundation, October 2006).

51 Milligan et al., "Turning Medicaid Beneficiaries into Purchasers of Health Care."

52 National Center for Policy Analysis, "Consumer Driven Health Care," *NCPA Study No. 288,* September 28, 2006, http://www.ncpa.org/pub/st/st288/st288g.html.

53 Agency for Health Care Administration (ACHA), *Florida Medicaid Reform: Application for 1115 Research and Demonstration Waiver* (Agency for Health Care Reform, August 30, 2006), l, fdhc.state.fl.us/Medicaid/medicaid_reform/waiver/pdfs/medical_reform_waiver_final_101905.pdf.

54 Ibid., 3.

55 Quoted in Nina Owcharenko and Robert Moffit, "The Massachusetts Health Plan: Lessons for the States," The Heritage Foundation, *Backgrounder No. 1953,* July 18, 2006, 1.

56 David Hyman, "The Massachusetts Health Plan: The Good, the Bad, and the Ugly," *Policy Analysis No. 595* (Washington, DC: Cato Institute, June 28, 2007).

57 Robert Moffit and Nina Owcharenko, "Understanding Key Parts of the Massachusetts Health Plan," WebMemo #1045, The Heritage Foundation, April 20, 2006.

58 Ibid.

59 Medicare Board of Trustees, *Status of the Social Security and Medicare Programs: A Summary of the 2006 Annual Reports*, http://www.ssa.gov/OACT/TRSUM/trsummary .html.

60 Robin Toner, "Gingrich Vows Total Review of Medicare for Cost Savings," *New York Times*, January 31, 1995, 1A.

61 Peter J. Ferrara, "Gingrich Can Avert GOP Disaster over Medicare," *Wall Street Journal*, May 9, 1995, A20.

62 Robert Pear, "Medicare Audits Show Problems in Private Plans," *New York Times*, October 7, 2007, http://query.nytimes.com/gst/fullpage.html?res=9F05E5D9133CF 934A35753CIA9619C8B63.

63 Michael Cannon and Michael D. Tanner, *Healthy Competition: What's Holding Back Health Care and How to Free It* (Washington, DC: The Cato Institute, 2005).

64 Pamela Herd, "Universalism Without the Targeting: Privatizing the Old Age Welfare State," *The Gerontologist* 45 (2005): 292–98.

65 Quoted in Dreyfuss and Stone, "Medikill," 2.

66 Joseph P. Newhouse, *Free for All? Lessons from the RAND Health Insurance Experiment* (Cambridge, MA: Harvard University Press, 1993).

67 Malcolm Gladwell, "The Moral-Hazard Myth: The Bad Idea Behind Our Failed Health Care System," *The New Yorker*, August 8, 2005, 1–10.

68 Kaiser Family Foundation, *Massachusetts Health Care Reform Plan* (Menlo Park, CA: Henry J. Kaiser Family Foundation, April 2006).

69 Kenneth E. Thorpe, "The Rise in Health Care Spending and What To Do About It," *Health Affairs* 24 (2005): 1436–45.

70 David Cutler, *Your Money or Your Life: Strong Medicine for America's Health Care System* (New York: Oxford University Press, 2004).

71 Timothy S. Jost, "Consumer-Driven Health Care in South Africa: Lessons from Comparative Health Policy Studies," *Journal of Health and Biomedical Law* 1 (2005): 83–109.

72 Tim Harford, *The Undercover Economist: Exposing Why the Rich are Rich, The Poor are Poor—and Why You Can Never Buy a Decent Used Car* (New York: Oxford University Press, 2006).

73 W. Von Eiff, T. Massaro, Y. O. Voo, and R. Ziegenbein, "Medical Savings Accounts:

A Core Feature of Singapore's Health Care System," *European Journal of Health Economics* 3 (2002): 188–95.

74 Jill Quadagno, "Why the United States Has No National Health Insurance: Stakeholder Mobilization Against the Welfare State, 1945–1996," *Journal of Health and Social Behavior* 45 (2004): 25–44. See also Quadagno, *One Nation, Uninsured*.

75 Health Insurance Association of America, http://www.ahip.org/.

76 American Medical Association, *Individual Responsibility to Obtain Health Insurance*, Report 3 of the Council on Medical Service, Resolution 703, 1-05, Reference Committee A, June 2006.

77 Ben Werner, "Blue Cross Banks on Health Savings Plans," *The State*, March 2, 2007, http://www.thestate.com/mid/thestate/business/16812989.

78 Kaiser Family Foundation, *National Survey of Enrollees*.

CHAPTER TWO

Uninsured in America:
New Realities, New Risks

KATHERINE SWARTZ

Why is it so important to have health insurance? It prevents financial ruin and provides access to medical care that leads to better health outcomes, especially if a person has a chronic disease such as cancer or an accident requiring expensive care.

This answer is less obvious than it sounds since it is often assumed that people without health insurance can get the same medical care as insured people. As President Bush said in a speech on July 10, 2007: "I mean, people have access to health care in America. After all, you just go to an emergency room."[1] What the president did not say, and what most people do not realize, is that all the hospitals are required to do by law is stabilize a patient. They do not have to provide further diagnostic tests or care for chronic conditions. Further, as Elizabeth Warren and Deborah Thorne detail in Chapter 3, when people are uninsured, they often face mounting debts for care that they would not have if they had insurance—and those debts can drive them into bankruptcy.

In 2006, 47 million Americans did not have any type of health insurance. This was 2.2 million more people than in 2005,[2] and it was the largest one-year increase in the number of uninsured since the Census Bureau started collecting insurance status data in 1979. Moreover, among people younger than sixty-five, the increase in the uninsured means that one in six nonelderly people (almost 18 percent) are now uninsured—and at risk for financial problems, receiving less care, and having poorer quality outcomes if they do need medical care.

There are three sections to this chapter. In the first, I discuss why it is so important for people to have health insurance and then describe who the uninsured are, with special attention to the largest subgroups of the uninsured. It is useful to have mental images of the types of people who are most likely to be without health insurance coverage. I then turn in the second section to the principal reasons so many people are uninsured: insurers' concerns that a disproportionate share of the people applying for individual coverage will have high medical costs, and the rising costs of medical care and health insurance. Understanding why people are increasingly without insurance is essential for devising policies that can significantly reduce the number of uninsured. Moreover, the rapidly rising costs of medical care and insurance are a warning that many people with insurance coverage are at risk of losing it. Thus, in the third section I examine two possible routes to universal coverage. One addresses the reasons people are currently uninsured and assumes that employer-sponsored health insurance will continue to cover a majority of people. The other, long-term route involves a restructuring of how we finance health insurance and how we might organize the purchasing of it if we want to have a choice of health plans. In the longer term, the growth in health care spending also must be slowed; this can occur if everyone has a basic level of health insurance that only covers medical services that are judged cost-effective. Finally, I conclude with a discussion about how to judge proposals to extend health insurance coverage and two hurdles facing proposals to reform the system of health insurance in the United States.

THE SCOPE OF THE PROBLEM OF BEING UNINSURED

The extent of the uninsured problem has at least two dimensions. One relates to the significant and negative consequences for people of being without health insurance. The other concerns the number of people without any type of coverage and the primary groups of people who are uninsured.

There are both financial and health-related consequences of being uninsured. Uninsured people are at risk for substantial sums of money to pay for unexpected medical care—and sometimes these bills are a financial catastrophe, causing many to declare bankruptcy (see chapter by Warren and Thorne). Even among people who do not declare bankruptcy, the fall-out from medical bills for emergency room visits or hospitalizations can have long-term consequences. Ironically, these outcomes include the depletion of savings and not being able to afford health insurance because the people are paying down debts that they would not have incurred had they been covered by health insurance.[3]

There is mounting evidence that not having insurance has negative effects on people's use of health care and on their health outcomes.[4] In a study of people who experienced a health shock (caused by an unintentional injury or the onset of a chronic condition), uninsured individuals were less likely to obtain any medical care and were more likely not to have received any recommended follow-up care than insured individuals.[5] Moreover, the uninsured with new chronic conditions reported significantly worse short-term health changes about 3.5 months after the initial shock and those who had an unintentional injury were significantly more likely to report that they were not fully recovered and were no longer being treated compared to those with health insurance.[6] A recent study conducted by the American Cancer Society shows that uninsured people are significantly less likely to get screened for cancer, more likely to be diagnosed with an advanced stage of the disease, and less likely to survive that diagnosis than their privately insured counterparts.[7] A similar study of people with diabetes underscored the importance of health insurance for receiving needed care and effectively managing the disease—many of the uninsured diabetics interviewed for the study had serious medical complications that likely would not have occurred had they been covered by insurance.[8]

Studies of people fifty to sixty-four years of age show that those who are uninsured receive fewer clinical services, are more likely to experience health declines, and die at younger ages than insured adults in the same age group.[9] When these uninsured individuals enrolled in Medicare at age sixty-five, they had greater use of health care and had higher medical spending than previously insured adults with similar characteristics at ages fifty-nine to sixty and comparable health insurance after age sixty-five.[10]

Thus, being uninsured has significant negative effects on people's financial situation and their use of health care and health outcomes. This is increasingly worrisome as the newer, more effective treatments for cancers and neurological chronic conditions involve pharmacological options that frequently are not offered to uninsured people. Similarly, uninsured people who have traumatic injuries from car or other accidents are far less likely to receive the continuum of care needed to make timely and good recoveries. All in all, being uninsured is dangerous for one's health.

ESTIMATING WHO IS UNINSURED AND MAJOR SUBGROUPS OF THE UNINSURED

As noted earlier, 47 million people were uninsured in 2006, and 46.4 million of them were under the age of sixty-five. These estimates are based on responses by a large, nationally representative sample of people who were asked by the census in March 2007 about their health insurance coverage in the previous calendar year.[11] Because the survey does not specifically capture times when people are uninsured for part of the year, the estimate of 47 million uninsured does not fully account for all the people who were affected by the lack of insurance during 2006.[12] Since the risks of being uninsured are large even for people who are uninsured for short periods of time, the annual census data provide a lower-bound estimate of the number of people affected by not having health insurance during a year. I follow the convention of relying on the annual census data to describe the uninsured rather than surveys that follow people over longer periods of time. The longer surveys have smaller samples of people, making estimates of subgroups of the uninsured less reliable, and the dynamics of health insurance coverage complicate analyses of the characteristics of the uninsured.

The characteristics of people who are most likely to be uninsured have changed over the past three decades. In the second section below, where I discuss the primary reasons people are uninsured, I explain why the types of people who are uninsured have changed. In this section, I describe the uninsured in terms of the largest subgroups among them. Three characteristics stand out as key predictors of who is uninsured:

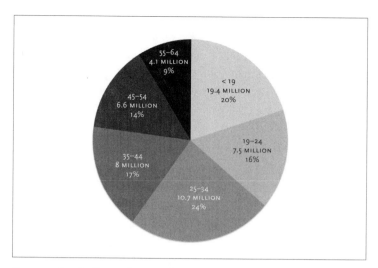

Figure 2.1   Age distribution of uninsured, 2006

being a younger adult twenty-five to forty-four years of age, having less formal education, and having low income.

ADULTS TWENTY-FIVE TO FORTY-FOUR YEARS OF AGE As can be seen in Figure 2.1, two out of five uninsured are twenty-five to forty-four years old. (By comparison, this age group accounts for not quite a third of the population under age sixty-five.) More significantly, the percents of all people in these age cohorts who are uninsured are at all-time highs: more than a quarter of all twenty-five- to thirty-four-year-olds and nearly a fifth of all thirty-five- to forty-four-year-olds were uninsured in 2006 (see Figure 2.2). These fractions of each cohort are twice what they were in 1979, when the census first started compiling annual data about health insurance.[13]

LESS FORMAL EDUCATION Almost two-thirds of uninsured adults twenty-three to sixty-four years of age have not gone past high school for formal education (see Figure 2.3). Having low levels of formal education is a large handicap for finding a job with employer-sponsored insurance (ESI): among adults who have not completed high school, 44 percent are uninsured; and a quarter of all adults who have high school diplomas but no further formal education are uninsured. These high fractions reflect

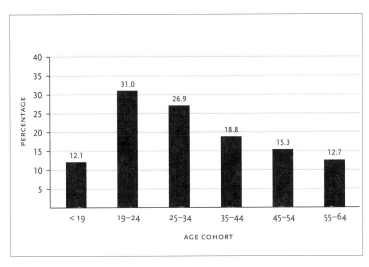

Figure 2.2   Fraction of people without health insurance by age cohort, 2006

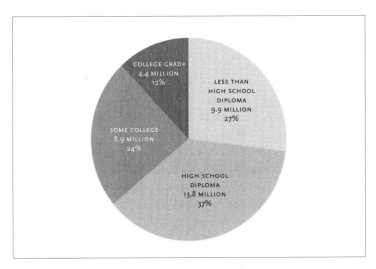

Figure 2.3   Education of uninsured adults 19 to 64 years of age, 2006

the decline in employer willingness to offer ESI and the fact that demand for people with less education is now largely in lower-wage jobs. This is a shift from a generation ago when high school graduates could find

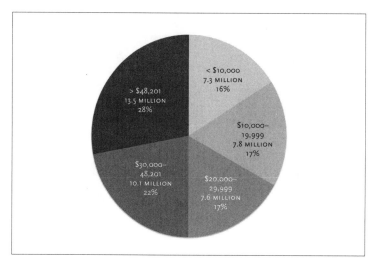

Figure 2.4 Family income of the nonelderly uninsured, 2006

well-paying jobs with large manufacturers. In 2006, five of the eight occupations that had the largest numbers of workers did not have high education requirements and more than a fifth of the people in each of these occupations were uninsured.

LOW INCOME As Figure 2.4 shows, 50 percent of the uninsured had family incomes below $30,000. (In contrast, only 26 percent of the population under age sixty-five had incomes below $30,000.) If we compare the incomes of the uninsured to the federal poverty level ($10,294 for an individual; $16,079 for a family of three; $20,614 for a family of four in 2006), a quarter of all the uninsured were officially in poverty in 2006. Another 29 percent had incomes between the poverty level and two times the poverty level (that is, they were near poor). Thus, 50 to 55 percent of the uninsured have low incomes (below $30,000 or below two times the poverty level) and cannot afford to purchase health insurance. In spite of the widespread (and mistaken) view that Medicaid covers all people in poverty, 34 percent of people with incomes below the poverty level were uninsured. Among all people who were near poor, 30 percent were uninsured.

Three other characteristics also describe significant but smaller subgroups among the uninsured: being middle class, being less than nineteen years old, and being foreign-born.

MIDDLE CLASS Being uninsured is not just a problem for low-income people—it also is increasingly a risk for middle-class people. The threshold level of income for the middle class can be defined as the median household income (that is, the income level at which 50 percent of all households in the country have incomes below it). In 2006, the median household income was $48,201, so anyone with an income above $48,201 can be defined as being in the middle class.[14] As Figure 2.4 shows, by this definition, 13.5 million of the 46.4 million nonelderly uninsured were middle class—29 percent of the uninsured. If we look just at working-age adults (twenty-three to sixty-four years old) who are also middle class, one in ten was uninsured in 2006. This is a significant change from 1979 when just 6 percent of middle-class adults were uninsured.

CHILDREN UNDER AGE NINETEEN In 2006, 9.4 million children were uninsured—an increase of 700,000 over the previous year. The increase in the number of uninsured children appears to be due to a drop in the number of children with access to employer-sponsored coverage—either because the parent lost access to employer coverage or because the employer raised the out-of-pocket cost of dependent coverage. In 2006, 63.4 percent of all children under age nineteen were covered by private insurance (employer sponsored or direct purchased) and 24.6 percent had public coverage (Medicaid or SCHIP, the State Children's Health Insurance Program). The fraction of all children who were uninsured was 12.1 percent, which was a slight increase over the last few years. Still, the fraction is significantly lower than it was in 1979 when 17 percent of all children were uninsured.[15]

Between the late 1980s and 2005, the number of uninsured children and the fraction of all children who were uninsured declined steadily—primarily because eligibility criteria for Medicaid were expanded to include older children at higher income levels and in 1997, the State Children's Health Insurance Program (SCHIP) was created.[16] States now have the option of covering children under Medicaid if their family incomes are as much as 185 percent of the poverty level. Uninsured children are eligible for SCHIP if their families have incomes that are too high for Medicaid but below a level set by each state. As of 2007, forty-one states and the District of Columbia had SCHIP income eligibility caps at or above 200 percent of the poverty level. SCHIP funding has included monies for outreach efforts, which have been credited with enrolling large numbers of children eligible for SCHIP and Medicaid.

Many analysts believe that without the increases in the Medicaid income eligibility limits for children and the implementation of SCHIP, the fraction of all children without health insurance would not have declined since 1979.[17] But there is a "chicken and egg" aspect to the decline in the rate of uninsured children. Some analysts argue that because more children are eligible for Medicaid and SCHIP, many employers no longer offer dependent coverage or have substantially increased the employee share of the premium for family coverage, effectively encouraging low-income workers to enroll their children in SCHIP.[18] However, case studies of SCHIP enrollment in specific states have found very few children who had ESI prior to enrolling in SCHIP and only a small fraction have a parent with ESI.[19] Thus, while in theory public programs may provide employers with an excuse to drop dependent coverage — what is known as the crowd-out effect — there is little evidence that this has occurred.

FOREIGN-BORN STATUS Just over a fifth of the uninsured in 2006 — ten million people — were not born in the United States and were not citizens. Another 2.3 million uninsured were foreign-born and were naturalized citizens. Not quite half (46.6 percent) of the foreign-born population who were not yet citizens was uninsured. This is in contrast to 15 percent of Americans born in the United States and 19.8 percent of naturalized citizens who were uninsured.

People who report themselves as foreign-born but not citizens on the census data are almost all here legally. Illegal immigrants are very unlikely to answer census survey questions. Thus, the foreign-born who are not citizens include people who have not yet lived here long enough to apply for citizenship and people who may expect to return to their country of origin some time in the future. Foreign-born residents who have been in the United States for longer periods of time are less likely to be uninsured than people who immigrated within the past five years.

A majority of foreign-born noncitizens are younger adults with low levels of formal education, who earn low wages — and do not have ESI at their jobs. But even middle-class and well-educated foreign-born noncitizens are more likely to be uninsured than their native-born counterparts. Although almost 40 percent of noncitizen residents have middle-class incomes, more than a quarter of them are uninsured.

It is too simple to say that most of the increase in the number of uninsured over the last two decades is due to the rising number of immigrants or that the number has increased because a large share of immigrants from Latin America (the origin of half the foreign-born population in 2000) lack formal education past the ninth grade or beyond high school.[20] Instead, the growth in the number of less educated immigrants in the past twenty years has to be seen as contributing to the imbalance between the demand for and supply of unskilled workers, enabling firms to hire low-wage workers without offering ESI.

UNDERINSURED PEOPLE In addition to the major groups of people without any health insurance, there are a substantial number of people who are underinsured—that is, although they have health insurance, it is not adequate in terms of protecting them against catastrophic medical expenses. People can be underinsured for a variety of reasons, including that they have out-of-pocket medical expenses that exceed 10 percent of income (or 5 percent of income for a low-income person, with income below 200 percent of the poverty level), or deductibles that are greater than 5 percent of income. A recent analysis of people with health insurance policies estimates that sixteen million adults nineteen to sixty-four years of age were underinsured in 2003.[21] As more people have health policies with annual deductibles upwards of $5,000, the number of underinsured is sure to increase. The underinsured are sheltered from some medical care costs, but since they are not protected against catastrophic costs they face the same financial and health risks as the uninsured.

PRINCIPAL REASONS PEOPLE ARE UNINSURED

DECLINE IN EMPLOYER-SPONSORED HEALTH INSURANCE —
AND A SIGNAL SHIFT IN EMPLOYER ATTITUDES ABOUT ESI

The large increase in the number of uninsured between 2005 and 2006 reflects a now almost decade-old decline in the percentage of people with ESI. In 2000, 68.3 percent of the population younger than sixty-five years of age had employer-sponsored coverage; in 2006, the fraction was 62.9 percent.[22] During this same time period, there was a steady decline in the fraction of firms that sponsor health insurance (from 69 percent in 2000 to 61 pecent in 2006).[23] In practice, the shrinking of ESI coverage is greater than these statistics suggest. Many firms that offer ESI to "regular" employees are increasingly using workers hired through contract houses (often known as contract workers) and temp agencies, and other self-employed people who work on specific tasks for long periods of time. When companies hire people in these ways, the workers are not technically employees and are not included in the fringe benefit plans the firms offer.[24] Younger adults are particularly likely to be employed as contract workers, which helps explain their significant representation among the uninsured.

Employer attitudes toward the costs of ESI reflect the labor markets in which they hire workers. Most of the growth in employment over the last two decades has been in the services sector, in particular health care services, professional business services, and leisure-hospitality-entertainment services. Many of the companies in these industries are small and employ large numbers of low-wage, less skilled workers. Immigrant labor is particularly prevalent in these occupational labor markets. As long as the supply of workers willing to work in these service jobs is much larger than the demand for them, the firms can keep wages low—and not offer ESI to attract or retain the workers. Moreover, the demand for the services provided by these industries is very price sensitive so firms are not in a position to charge higher prices in order to provide higher wages and ESI.

The decline in the proportion of firms offering ESI and the increased use of contract workers are warning signs that it is unlikely that ESI will continue to cover a majority of Americans. These signs indicate the extent to which companies are moving to limit their financial risk of increases in health care costs over which they do not have direct control. For employers, the fastest rising labor cost has been health insurance. Since 1996, premiums for ESI (both actual policies purchased from insurers and premium-equivalent costs for self-insured plans) have grown every year; the increases reflect the doubling of health care spending since 1996. Between 2001 and 2007, premiums for firms with more than three employees increased 78 percent—outpacing general inflation, which rose 17 percent.[25]

These premium increases occurred in spite of most employers shifting more out-of-pocket costs onto the workers in the form of higher deductibles and co-payments, and implementing more restrictions on pharmaceuticals and mental health benefits. These cost-shifting moves helped reduce the rate at which premiums rose but they also shifted more medical care costs onto people who became sick. In addition, although the average shares of premiums paid by employees (16% for single policies and 28% for family policies) have remained constant since 1999, there is some evidence to suggest that workers paying the highest shares are those with lower incomes.[26] A major survey of ESI premiums recently found that workers in firms with a high proportion of low-wage workers (35 percent or more of workers earn less than $21,000 a year) pay a higher share of family policy premiums than do workers in firms with lower proportions of low-wage workers.[27] Although the rate of increase in premiums between 2006 and 2007 (6.1 percent) was the smallest since 1999, it was still double the general rate of inflation.

Companies' willingness to sponsor group coverage is increasingly strained by the fact that health insurance costs have been rising faster than inflation and labor productivity. In a world of increased global competition, firms are moving to reduce their financial exposure to costs over which they have little control—and health insurance is high on that list. Policy analysts have long focused on small firms because a much smaller fraction of them offer ESI to their employees compared with large firms; for example, only 36 percent of firms with less than ten employees offer ESI while 95 percent of firms with more than one hundred employees do.[28] But now large firms are raising questions about how much they should be contributing toward health insurance. The CEO of General Motors, Rick Wagoner, has suggested that most of the costs of people with catastrophic medical expenses should be shifted to a federal government program, much like the costs of a natural disaster have become a federal responsibility. This shift in large companies' attitudes toward the cost of ESI, which comes on top of the increased use of temporary and contract workers in order to avoid including them in fringe benefits, deserves attention. It indicates that ESI as we have known it is not something to be counted on in the future.

HIGH PREMIUMS FOR INDIVIDUAL (NONGROUP) INSURANCE — COUNTERING THE RISK OF ADVERSE SELECTION

People who do not have access to ESI have only one choice for purchasing health insurance: the individual insurance market in their state—the market in which insurers sell policies covering individuals (and their dependents) rather than policies covering groups of people. Individual insurance is far more expensive than ESI because insurers face the risk that a disproportionate number of people who want to purchase individual policies are at higher risk of having high medical costs than the general population. This risk is known as adverse selection. As a result, premiums for individual policies can cost between $100 and $400 per month depending on a person's age and which state he or she lives in, and the less expensive policies come with a deductible of $1,000 or $2,000; premiums for family policies typically cost more than $700 per month and have a deductible of $5,000 or more.

In spite of the fact that many younger adults do not have ESI and are good candidates to purchase individual coverage, the rise in health care costs has driven up both premiums and the risk of adverse selection in the individual market. There is a catch-22 vicious cycle about this. Increasingly, the people who purchase individual insurance are forty-five and older — ages when health care spending tends to increase. It is not uncommon for those who are older or have medical conditions to face premiums in the individual market of $12,000 or more per year or to be offered policies that do not include care related to their conditions. Those who are younger and healthy also generally face premiums that are high relative to what they think their health care costs are likely to be because insurers expect that adverse selection is occurring also among the younger adults. The result is that individual policies are unattractive and unaffordable to younger adults. Even those who are earning middle-class incomes may decide that any "normal" medical care they might use would cost less than the premiums they would face in the individual market.

UNAFFORDABILITY OF HEALTH INSURANCE FOR LOWER INCOME PEOPLE

In addition to individual market policies being generally quite expensive, almost half of the uninsured (22.8 million) are people with annual incomes below $30,000. Among these low-income uninsured are 4.4 million children, many of whom may be eligible for Medicaid and SCHIP. Some of the 18.4 million uninsured adults with incomes below $30,000 may have access to ESI but the evidence is that only a small fraction of people (around 3 percent) who are offered ESI turn it down and are uninsured.[29] But most likely, the reason most of these lower income people are uninsured is that they do not have access to ESI and simply cannot afford to purchase insurance in the nongroup market. Premiums upwards of $8,000 per year for family policies on incomes of $30,000 or less would account for more than a quarter of the family's income—a fraction that most of us would consider totally unaffordable.

HOW CAN WE REDUCE THE NUMBER OF UNINSURED?

There is no single best strategy for how to reduce the number of uninsured and move toward universal coverage in the United States. This goal can be accomplished in a number of ways. Clearly, it will require political leadership and a belief among many different stakeholders that they will benefit if there is a significant reduction in the number of uninsured. Policymakers in both the public and private sectors are going to have to negotiate and make compromises to arrive at a strategy for achieving universal coverage. But it is essential that the strategy address the primary reasons people have trouble obtaining coverage: lack of access to employer-sponsored coverage, and the risk of adverse selection in the individual and small-group markets. Adverse selection is what causes premiums to be relatively high in the individual and small-group markets and especially unaffordable to people with low incomes. In what follows, I examine two possible routes to universal coverage. One route has a near-term time horizon; it addresses the reasons people are currently uninsured and assumes that employer-sponsored health insurance will continue to cover a majority of people. The other route involves a major, long-term restructuring of how we finance health insurance and how we might organize the purchasing of it if we want to continue to have a choice of health plans. This second course of action responds to the increasing possibility that a significant share of employers will limit their financial contributions to employee health insurance.

NEAR-TERM ROUTE

EXPAND PUBLIC PROGRAMS TO COVER ALL POOR AND NEAR POOR As noted earlier, a quarter of the uninsured—11.5 million people—had incomes below the poverty level in 2006. They represent a third of all poor people; a major share of the poor who do have health coverage are covered by Medicaid and a small share have ESI. Most of the uninsured in poverty are children whose parents have not enrolled them in Medicaid (for which they are eligible) and adults who are not eligible for Medicaid and do not have ESI. Uninsured people with incomes below the poverty level simply cannot afford to purchase health insurance on their own. They will be insured only if a public program is created to cover them or if Medicaid eligibility is expanded to include them.

Another 13.6 million of the uninsured (29 percent) are near poor, with incomes between one and two times the poverty level. Most people with incomes below two times the poverty level live in families with no more than three people, so $32,000 is approximately the top income for most of the near poor. Near poor uninsured adults generally have hourly wages not much above the minimum wage ($10 per hour is equivalent to $20,000 per year if a person works a forty-hour week for fifty weeks). People with incomes below $32,000 cannot afford to buy family coverage in the individual market; and anyone who has had a health problem in the past or who is between forty-five and sixty-four years of age is highly likely to be rejected for coverage or to face individual premiums of more than $1,000 per month. Thus, the only way they will gain coverage is if there is a public health coverage program or a highly subsidized program that involves private insurance plans. For example, a highly subsidized program like SCHIP that involves private insurance plans might be attractive to near-poor people even if they had to pay a nominal premium to enroll.

There are another 9.2 million uninsured (almost 20 percent of the uninsured) with incomes between two and three times the poverty level. Many of these lower income people, particularly those with incomes closer to two times the poverty level, will be unlikely to purchase coverage on their own without substantial subsidies. But if those subsidies were linked with other strategies (including reinsurance and pooling mechanisms, discussed below) to reduce premiums and increase access to health insurance choices, it seems likely that many of these 9.2 million people (7.4 million adults and 1.8 million children) could afford to buy coverage.

USE TAX CREDITS TO SUBSIDIZE PEOPLE WHO DO NOT HAVE ACCESS TO ESI AND BUY POLICIES IN THE INDIVIDUAL INSURANCE MARKETS People who do not have access to ESI where they work and are not self-employed are not eligible for a tax subsidy of their premium payments. This is in direct contrast to the tax code subsidization of health insurance for people who have ESI or are self-employed. People whose employers offer ESI do not pay payroll or income taxes on the share of premiums that employers pay.[30] Similarly, people who are self-employed may deduct the full amount of the premium they pay for health insurance from their income (so long as the premium does not exceed the income) before determining their income tax. This means that the self-employed are able to buy health insurance with pretax income (that is, income that is not subject to income or payroll taxes). Thus, there is a large tax advantage in receiving part of compensation in the form of employer contributions to health insurance premiums or being self-employed and purchasing health insurance.

The tax code treatment of employer payments for health insurance reduced federal revenues by more than $200 billion in fiscal year 2007.[31] (As a point of comparison, the revenues foregone by the tax code subsidy for ESI amount to more than the federal government's share of Medicaid expenses in fiscal year 2007.) Moreover, the tax code subsidization of ESI is more valuable to higher income people because at higher incomes, the marginal income tax rate is higher; not having to pay that tax on the employer share of ESI provides a large subsidy. When the tax subsidy is taken into account, the Tax Policy Center of the Urban Institute and the Brookings Institution estimates that the after-tax premium is on average equal to 6.8 percent of income for all tax units that have health coverage — but it is less than this for all tax units with incomes above $100,000.[32] Anyone with an income between $200,000 and $500,000, for example, is estimated to have an after-tax premium of only 2.7 percent of income, while someone with an income between $30,000 and $40,000 has an after-tax premium equal to 13.9 percent of income.

We could extend this tax advantage to anyone who does not have access to ESI and is not self-employed but earns enough to pay income taxes. The simplest form of this strategy consists of tax credits, where a person's taxes are reduced by some amount of money if the person purchases health insurance. One version of tax credits would have individuals receive a $1,000 credit and families a $2,500 credit for purchasing coverage. In his 2007 State of the Union speech, President Bush went much farther — he proposed abolishing the current tax code treatment of ESI and replacing it with a tax credit system of $7,500 for individuals and $15,000 for families.[33] The advantage of tax credits over permitting people to deduct the premium from their income is that tax credits do not encourage people to buy overly generous policies; tax credits are the same for people regardless of which policy they buy.

Many people would not be able to take advantage of tax credits, however. People who earn low incomes and therefore owe little or no income tax cannot take a credit for more than the taxes they owe — the net premium they would face is almost the full premium. People with lower middle-class incomes might take advantage of the tax credits to purchase insurance if they were able to receive a portion of the credit each month or a twelfth of the credit could be sent each month to an insurance plan. The practical problem with setting up a monthly allotment of a health insurance tax credit is that it requires a person to have an employer who will then add the allotment to the person's wages or send it to an insurance company. Since many people without access to ESI work for small firms, the firms will not be able to provide the additional funds to their workers or the health plans unless the firms receive the funds throughout the year. These problems could be addressed if we wanted to create a tax credit subsidy of health insurance purchases by people without access to ESI. But the most efficient way to subsidize the purchase of private health insurance by lower income people would be to provide a direct subsidy that declines as a person's income rises.

It is doubtful, moreover, that just offering tax credit subsidies to people without access to ESI will substantially increase the number of people who buy health insurance. The tax deductibility of premiums for the self-employed has not significantly increased the number of self-employed who purchase coverage.[34] Even with the tax deduction for self-employed people, premiums in the individual market are relatively high and the tax deduction cannot be taken until income taxes are filed. Thus, tax credits would need to be put in place with strategies that could reduce insurers' concern with adverse selection and thereby reduce premiums.

REDUCE THE RISK OF ADVERSE SELECTION As noted earlier, a major reason premiums are high in the small-group and individual insurance markets is that there is a potential for adverse selection in those markets. Since the risk of adverse selection is what causes insurers to charge high rates in the small-group and individual markets, strategies are needed to reduce the risk to insurers of having a disproportionate number of very-high-cost enrollees.

One such strategy involves three policies that would work best if they were jointly implemented: merge the small-group and individual markets; create a government-sponsored reinsurance program to spread the costs of people with the very highest medical costs among all taxpayers; and require everyone to purchase a minimum level of health insurance.

Merge small-group and individual markets In most states, the number of people with small-group insurance is substantially larger than the number with individual coverage.[35] This is consistent with insurers' concerns that the individual market is a high-risk market where young, healthy people do not purchase coverage. The result is that premiums are particularly high in the individual market, providing a further disincentive for young and healthy people to buy policies.

The distinction between the small-group and individual insurance markets has its origins in the early 1900s. Although the distinction seemed meaningful for part of the twentieth century, it seems less so now as a growing number of people work for small firms that do not offer ESI and more people are self-employed workers. In earlier years, many of these people would have been covered through small-group policies but now their only option for purchasing coverage is through the individual markets. If the two types of markets were to be merged in each of the states, the combined market might raise premiums a small amount for workers in small firms that already offer ESI but it also would reduce premiums for individuals.

By itself, however, a policy of merging the individual and small-group markets may reduce premiums by only 10 to 15 percent for people who previously had to buy policies in the individual market.[36] Given what we know about how price sensitive people are when it comes to buying health insurance, a decline of 10 to 15 percent may not cause a significant number of uninsured individuals to purchase policies. Thus, a merger of these two markets needs to be one part of a multipart strategy to reduce adverse selection.

A government-sponsored reinsurance program for the small-group and individual markets A more direct way of addressing insurers' concern with adverse selection is to create a government-sponsored reinsurance program for the small-group and individual insurance markets.[37] Reinsurance is essentially insurance for insurers—either for the possibility that some individuals will have very expensive medical care or that a group of individuals will together have medical expenses above some threshold. The former type—known as excess-of-loss reinsurance—is particularly suited to addressing insurers' concern with adverse selection because it provides protection against the possibility that some individuals may have very high costs. A government-sponsored reinsurance program would pick up a large share (anywhere from 50 to 95 percent) of the costs for people who have annual medical spending that qualifies for the reinsurance. The reinsurance could cover people with medical costs in the top 1 or 2 percent of the population—or it could pick up a large share of individuals' annual costs in a limited slice (or corridor) of health care expenses, perhaps between $30,000 and $100,000, for example. Note that reinsurance does not cover all of the expenses above the threshold for when it kicks in; the original insurance plan is still responsible for a share of the costs. That share can be 50 or 10 or 5 percent, and it can have different values for different corridors of the distribution of health care spending. Because the original insurer retains responsibility for a share of a person's costs, it has a strong incentive to manage the care of the people who are very sick, thereby reducing unnecessary care and expenses.

Reinsurance would immediately bring down insurers' risk of having a disproportionate number of very-high-cost people. With less risk, the insurers can then lower the premiums. The Healthy New York program (restricted to people who have incomes below 250 percent of the poverty level or who work in small firms and earn less than $35,000) has premiums that are about half of what they are in the standard individual market in New York.[38] The premiums are much lower than might be expected on the basis of knowing that people in the top 1 percent of the medical expenditure distribution account for about 30 percent of all medical spending in the United States. The larger reduction in Healthy New York premiums seems to be because the risk to insurers of having a large number of people with very high costs is reduced by the reinsurance.

The biggest hurdle in considering a reinsurance program is its costs, especially if it were to cover almost all of the costs of people whose medical expenses put them in the top 1 or 2 percent of the population. The program costs could be reduced, however, if the reinsurance were structured to cover a particular slice of the costs of higher cost people or if the original insurer had responsibility for more than 5 percent of the costs. In

Healthy New York, for example, the reinsurance covers 90 percent of the annual costs of people whose expenses are between $5,000 and $75,000; expenses below $5,000 and above $75,000 are fully the responsibility of the HMO. There are many ways to structure a reinsurance program and the costs of various alternative structures could be estimated in order to choose one that balances a need to reduce premiums and be cost-effective. It also would be easier to administer a reinsurance program for a merged small group and individual market than for the two markets separately.

Require people to buy health insurance The third policy to reduce adverse selection is a requirement that everyone buy at least a minimum level of health insurance. (People with low incomes would be subsidized, as noted above.) The only way to reduce the threat of adverse selection for a market as a whole is to require that people purchase coverage. This is why insisting that people have at least a minimum level of health insurance is gaining attention among policymakers and the public—it is the surest way to bring younger, healthy people into the pool of people covered by policies sold in the small-group and individual insurance markets.

Requiring people to purchase at least a minimum health insurance policy has to be done in the context of a social compact between individuals and society: if everyone enrolls in an insurance plan and contributes to the overall insurance pool, then society will ensure that anyone who becomes very sick will receive medical care.[39] This social compact also requires that government ensure that affordable health insurance is available. This could be done by creating insurance pooling mechanisms that would allow people without access to ESI to obtain coverage that would have benefits and premiums similar to those that people in large employer groups enjoy. The Massachusetts' Commonwealth Connector is such a pooling mechanism; currently it offers a choice of four different insurers, each of which must offer four different plans. HealthPass in New York City is another pooling mechanism—it is for small businesses and was set up by the New York Business Group on Health, the City of New York, and the health insurance industry of New York.[40] Four insurers participate and offer a choice of thirty different health plans. In addition to the efficiencies gained from pooling, the pooling mechanisms offer advantages to employers and individuals. Employers can pay part of the premium but they do not have to be responsible for sponsoring the health plans offered to people. Individuals have a choice of plan options that must meet a minimum level of benefits and they cannot be turned down by their choice. The pooling mechanisms also can be set up such that employers can create accounts that allow workers to pay the premiums with pretax dollars.[41]

These near-term policies are useful for helping people who currently do not have health insurance. But they do not address the increasing threat that employers will limit their financial contributions to ESI and perhaps their role even in sponsoring group coverage to employees. I turn next to a second course of actions and policies that do that.

LONG-TERM RESTRUCTURING OF FINANCING
AND ORGANIZING HEALTH INSURANCE

Since the early 1980s, American companies have been facing increasingly competitive world markets. As a result, relative labor costs have become an issue for most companies — and since health insurance costs are rising faster than labor productivity, they catch companies' attention. Further, health insurance costs are not something employers can control. Even though most large companies (those with more than five hundred employees) self-insure their employees' and dependents' medical costs, the growth in health care spending is driven by factors that even insurance companies have difficulty controlling. It is not surprising then that companies are beginning to say that they want to limit their financial exposure to future increases in medical costs. So far, they have moved to increase the cost-sharing required of employees but it is increasingly clear that many companies would like to abandon sponsorship of health benefits altogether. If the tax code were altered to limit how employer contributions to premiums were treated or if everyone were given a tax credit for purchasing insurance as the Bush administration proposed, it is likely that many companies would stop offering ESI.

The shift in companies' attitudes about their role in offering ESI offers an opportunity for rethinking how we might achieve universal coverage. In particular, we need to plan for major changes in how health insurance is financed and how people could obtain coverage.

RESTRUCTURE FINANCING OF HEALTH INSURANCE Two principles should be put forth at the outset of considering how we might restructure the financing of health insurance in the United States. First, employers gain great benefits from having both a healthy workforce and a healthy pool of potential workers. Because of this, employers and companies should continue to pay part of health insurance costs in the United States. Second, everyone should be in the new system so the financing will take account of the fact that lower income people cannot pay as much as higher income people. How the full cost of health insurance is divided up among individuals and companies, and among individuals by income, then depends on what we know about incentives embedded in various types of taxes and the distributional effects of different ways we might structure such taxes and premium payments.

Other countries have wrestled with how to structure the financing of their health insurance and they offer examples for the United States. In particular, several European Union countries have revised their health insurance systems within the last decade as part of their efforts to slow the growth in health care spending and in response to the EU's requirement that health insurance be portable across country borders. Most of the countries rely on a mix of individual and employer premiums or taxes to pay for the insurance, and many countries have a mix of private and public health insurance plan options. The Netherlands and Germany offer two examples.

The Netherlands altered its health insurance system just two years ago (January 2006). All adults pay a nominal premium (about 1050 euros in 2006, or about $1,500 using late 2007 exchange rates between the dollar and the euro) that depends on which of thirty-three private health plans the adult chooses.[42] In addition to the premium, employers pay a payroll tax of 6.5 percent on their employees' income up to 30,105 euros in 2006 (about $43,000)—or a maximum of about 2,000 euros ($2,900) per year.[43] Self-employed people and retirees pay 4.4 percent of their income. Low-income people can apply for a subsidy, which is dependent on a person's income; about 30 percent (5 million people) of the population receive such subsidies.

Germany requires that all people with annual incomes below about 47,250 euros ($67,570 using late 2007 exchange rates) participate in a public insurance system; about 10 percent of the population is exempt from the social system. The social system has a basic benefits package for which employees pay 7.5 percent of their salary (up to 47,250 euros) and employers pay 6.6 percent of their workers' salaries (up to 47,250 euros) for insurance. Children and nonworking spouses are covered "free of charge"; there are no distinctions between individual and family policies. However, in the private insurance system where people can purchase supplementary coverage (chiefly to cover private hospital rooms and perhaps greater choice of health care providers), family members are charged separately. Private insurance premiums are set to reflect the expected risk of individuals—and the insurance companies can turn down people for coverage (unlike the social insurance system).

The United States could restructure its financing of health insurance along lines similar to those used by the Netherlands, Germany, and others in the EU and the OECD. We could create a mix of financing sources that includes individual premiums and income-related taxes. The individual premiums could be relatively modest and would depend on which health plan was chosen. The income-related taxes could apply to all of a person's income or there could be a cap on the income which is taxable (as with the Social Security tax). Since we also want companies to contribute to the health insurance financing, companies could be required to pay a payroll tax that would be dedicated to health insurance. Such a financing structure also could be used to eliminate separate programs for the poor. In Europe, lower income people are offered the same choices at least for basic coverage as higher income people. Their payments are subsidized by higher income people and companies, but they are not shifted into a separate program like Medicaid.

REORGANIZE HOW WE CHOOSE HEALTH PLANS With employers less likely to sponsor health insurance, we will need an alternative arrangement for how we choose health insurance. Recall that in this new world of reorganizing how we finance health insurance and choose among health plans, everyone would be covered and the only difference in what anyone would pay would be the nominal per-person premium—which would depend on the health plan chosen. How we choose health insurance plans could still involve ESI; many employers may be willing to sponsor insurance options as a way of attracting and retaining employees. But for people who do not have employers that sponsor group policies, the pooling mechanisms described earlier would be the most efficient way of offering health plan options from which people could choose. The pooling mechanism agency would set standards for a minimum basic benefits package that every policy must cover and require insurers to accept all applicants. In exchange for requiring insurers to accept all applicants, the pooling agency also would establish an adjustment to the premium based on a person's "risk" of needing higher cost medical care so the health plans would not have an incentive to provide less than optimal care for high-cost people. The risk adjustment would be funded out of revenues raised by taxing individuals and companies. The Dutch have such a risk-adjustment system and risk-adjustment models have been used in conjunction with Medicare and Medicaid for more than a decade.

Given that not all health plans in the United States are national plans and that we have a strong tradition of state regulation of health insurance, it is likely that at least initially the pooling mechanisms would be created within a state or substate geographic regions (as with Northern and Southern California, or upstate and downstate New York or Illinois). However, because much of the funding for health insurance will be collected through the federal tax system, it will be necessary to have adjustments to the per-capita funds that are returned to the pooling agencies based on differences in costs of providing medical care across states and substate regions. Such adjustments could be done on a basis similar to that currently used to adjust Medicare payments to physicians and hospitals.

SLOW THE GROWTH IN HEALTH CARE SPENDING For the past decade, health care spending per capita and health insurance premiums have been rising faster than both general price inflation and productivity growth. The gulf between the growth in insurance costs and productivity is why many employers have opted out of sponsoring group health benefits and caused those that do offer ESI to increase employee cost sharing so workers may have more incentive to hold down health care spending. Although there may be benefits to the increased spending on health care,[44] it also is clear that health care cannot continue to absorb an ever-larger share of families' budgets or federal and state budgets. There are opportunity costs to spending on health—such spending is crowding out other priorities such as education, repairing and expanding infrastructure, and national security.

By the same logic, the United States will not be able to afford to provide everyone with a basic level of health insurance unless the growth in health care spending is brought under control. Two types of health care spending are driving the overall growth in spending. One type includes expensive but not super-high-cost diagnostic, surgical, and pharmaceutical services that are no longer considered high risk so more people are taking advantage of them, especially because insurance covers their costs. Hip replacements and chemotherapies for some cancers are examples of this driver of health care spending. The other type consists of very new and very expensive diagnostic and treatment options for cancers, chronic conditions, and acute traumas. New radiological scanning devices and new forms of radiation surgery such as the CyberKnife® are examples of the technical innovations that are capable of saving some people's lives. However, they are enormously expensive—and the money spent on such machines, as well as the teams of people needed to manage them, is money that cannot be used for other purposes.

To control the growth in health care spending, there will need to be limits on what medical services are included under basic health insurance coverage. As a society, we may want basic insurance to cover the first type of expensive services, especially since they improve the quality of life for large numbers of people. But the second type of health care spending raises issues of how far we want to go with basic insurance coverage. Cost-sharing mechanisms, such as deductibles and co-insurance or co-payments, can help make people think about the costs of health care but they have almost no effect on the treatment choices of people who are very sick and have expenses above $10,000 deductibles. Slowing the growth in health care spending ultimately will not be possible unless the basic benefits package excludes treatments that are enormously expensive and not cost-effective. A new and independent federal agency is needed to determine the cost-effectiveness of new diagnostic tests and medical therapies, and only those deemed cost-effective should be covered by the basic health plans. Limiting what basic health insurance pays for is unavoidable if we are to control health care spending.

As long as we do not have everyone covered by a basic level of health insurance, it is relatively easy for the health care system to face very few limits on what is covered by insurance. The result is what we have seen for the past four decades: an increasing fraction of the population without health insurance while those with insurance have both access to excellent health care and relatively low out-of-pocket expenses for such care. A new financing and organizational structure that ensures that everyone has basic health insurance would enable us to slow the growth in health care spending.

With 46.4 million people under age sixty-five uninsured and upwards of 30 million more either uninsured part of the year or underinsured, and companies increasingly resisting paying for increases in health spending that they cannot control, it is clear that the current system of health insurance in the United States is in trouble. Proposals for reforms need to address simultaneously the reasons people are uninsured and the fact that companies are no longer able to pay health insurance costs that grow faster than worker productivity.

Although the major criterion for judging reform proposals is how many people would be insured as a result of each, two additional sets of criteria also should be used to evaluate the proposals. One set centers on the major subgroups of the uninsured: Do the reforms make insurance affordable for younger adults and poor people? Do they address the adverse-selection risk that causes high premiums in the individual markets, leaving many middle-class people without ESI uninsured? Another set of criteria for judging reform proposals focuses on how they would restructure how we pay for health insurance and the distributional effects of the restructured financing.

Using the first set of criteria, only proposals that completely subsidize health insurance coverage for people with incomes below $30,000 (or below two times the poverty level) will ensure coverage for the poor and near poor. They cannot afford to purchase health insurance in the individual market, and if they have access to ESI, they are going to be uninsured unless the employee out-of-pocket cost of the premium is very low. Proposals built on employer mandates are unlikely to help many low-wage workers since most low-income people work for small firms (often with fewer than ten employees) that have low profit margins and cannot pay for ESI. Reforms focused on tax credits or subsidies to low-income people if they buy insurance in the individual market generally have offered small credits or subsidies relative to the premiums. The premiums still would be unaffordable to almost all low-income individuals and would cause very few to become insured.

Individual insurance markets can be an option for middle-class people only if the premiums are affordable. Premiums are high in these markets because insurers are concerned about the risk of adverse selection. Reform proposals have to address this risk for individual coverage to be affordable—particularly to young and healthy adults who do not have ESI. Proposals that require everyone to have health insurance (with appropriate subsidies) would go far in reducing adverse selection and therefore premiums in the individual markets. Coupling such a requirement with a government-sponsored reinsurance program that shifts most of the expenses of the highest cost people to the broad population base also would address the adverse selection risk and significantly reduce premiums.

Proposals to help the uninsured also must take a longer term view of how health insurance is financed and organized. Given the pressures to reduce labor costs resulting from global competition, we cannot count on ESI to be the mainstay of our system of health insurance in the future.[45] Moreover, requiring companies to provide ESI without acknowledging the economic realities of the competition they are facing is not realistic. None of the current proposals for insurance reform includes plans for restructuring the financing and organization of health insurance.

Many policymakers and analysts believe the biggest hurdle to reforming the U.S. health insurance system is that providing a basic level of health insurance to everyone will require more money. To be sure, we already pay for the medical care of the uninsured when they seek care—care that often is expensive because it is provided in high-cost settings such as hospital emergency departments. One estimate is that the uninsured obtained $35 billion of uncompensated care in 2001, and that government spending (tax revenues) paid for 80 to 85 percent of that.[46] But when people have insurance coverage they generally use more medical care than the uninsured so there will be an increase in total health care spending if everyone has coverage. In spite of methodological differences across several different estimates of this increase, they all predict an increase of between 3 and 6 percent of total spending, or between $34 and $69 billion (in 2001 dollars).[47] These estimates indicate a relatively small additional cost of providing coverage to everyone.

The United States can afford to cover everyone with a basic health insurance policy. How we do so is the question facing us in the next decade. We need to start the political negotiations and discussions to get there—before many more millions of Americans lose health insurance.

APPENDIX

[Source: Author's analyses of the March 1980 and March 2007 Current Population Surveys]

AGE COHORT	1979 NUMBER OF UNINSURED (MILLIONS)	PERCENT OF UNINSURED	SIMPLE PROBABILITY OF BEING UNINSURED BY AGE COHORT	2006 NUMBER OF UNINSURED (MILLIONS)	PERCENT OF UNINSURED	SIMPLE PROBABILITY OF BEING UNINSURED BY AGE COHORT
< 19	10.784	39.3%	17.0%	9.438	20.3%	12.1%
19 to 24	4.974	18.1%	21.5%	7.540	16.2%	31.0%
25 to 34	4.112	15.0%	12.1%	10.710	23.1%	26.9%
35 to 44	2.438	8.9%	10.0%	8.016	17.3%	18.8%
45 to 54	2.349	8.5%	10.8%	6.640	14.3%	15.3%
55 to 64	2.818	10.3%	14.0%	4.094	8.8%	12.7%
TOTAL	27.47	100.1%	14.7%	46.438	100%	17.8%

Table 2.1   Ages of the nonelderly uninsured and simple probabilities of being uninsured by age cohort, 1979 and 2006

EDUCATION COHORT	1979 NUMBER OF UNINSURED (MILLIONS)	PERCENT OF UNINSURED	SIMPLE PROBABILITY OF BEING UNINSURED BY EDUCATION	2006 NUMBER OF UNINSURED (MILLIONS)	PERCENT OF UNINSURED	SIMPLE PROBABILITY OF BEING UNINSURED BY EDUCATION
DID NOT FINISH HIGH SCHOOL	5.768	34.9%	20.3%	9.863	26.7%	43.7%
HIGH SCHOOL GRADUATE	6.045	36.6%	12.0%	13.823	37.4%	24.8%
SOME COLLEGE/ ASSOC. DEGREE	3.087	18.7%	13.5%	8.924	24.1%	16.9%
COLLEGE GRAD./ POST-GRADUATE	1.629	9.9%	7.9%	4.389	11.9%	8.5%
TOTAL	16.529	100.1%	13.5%	37.000	101.1%	20.3%

Table 2.2   Education of uninsured adults nineteen to sixty-four years of age and simple probabilities of being uninsured by education cohort, 1979 and 2006

FAMILY INCOME GROUP (2006 $)	1979 NUMBER OF UNINSURED (MILLIONS)	PERCENT OF UNINSURED	SIMPLE PROBABILITY OF BEING UNINSURED BY INCOME GROUP	2006 NUMBER OF UNINSURED (MILLIONS)	PERCENT OF UNINSURED	SIMPLE PROBABILITY OF BEING UNINSURED BY INCOME GROUP
< $10,000	5.000	18.2%	38.8%	7.336	15.8%	35.7%
$10,000– 19,999	5.466	19.9%	29.2%	7.837	16.9%	34.4%
$20,000– 29,999	5.091	18.6%	22.8%	7.642	16.5%	30.5%
$30,000– 48,201	4.236	15.4%	13.9%	10.092	21.7%	21.8%
> $48,201	7.678	27.9%	7.6%	13.531	29.1%	9.3%
TOTAL	27.47	100%	14.7%	46.438	100%	17.8%

Table 2.3   Family income of the nonelderly uninsured and simple probabilities of being uninsured by income group, 1979 and 2006

NOTES

1 President Bush spoke at the Intercontinental Hotel in Cleveland, Ohio; the full speech is available at http://www.whitehouse.gov/news/releases/2007/07/20070 710-6.html.

2 Author's analysis of the *March Current Population Survey*, released by the U.S. Census Bureau, August 28, 2007.

3 Kaiser Commission on Medicaid and the Uninsured, *In Their Own Words: The Uninsured Talk About Living Without Health Insurance*, September 2000, www.kff.org/ uninsured/loader.cfm?url=/commonspot/security/getfile.cfm&PageID=13470.

4 See especially J. Hadley, "Sicker and Poorer: The Consequences of Being Uninsured," *Medical Care Research and Review* 60, no. 2 Supplement (2003): 3s–75s; and Institute of Medicine, *Care Without Coverage: Too Little, Too Late* (Washington, DC: National Academy Press, 2002).

5 J. Hadley, "Insurance Coverage, Medical Care Use, and Short-term Health Changes Following an Unintentional Injury or the Onset of a Chronic Condition," *JAMA* 297, no. 10 (2007): 1073–84.

6 Ibid.

7 E. Ward, M. Halpern, N. Schrag, V. Cokkinides, C. DeSantis, P. Bandi, R. Siegel, A. Stewart, and A. Jemal, "Association of Insurance with Cancer Care Utilization and Outcomes," *CA: A Cancer Journal for Clinicians* 58, no. 1 (2008) 9–31.

8 K. Pollitz, E. Bangit, K. Lucia, M. Kofman, K. Montgomery, and H. Whelan, *Falling Through the Cracks: Stories of How Health Insurance Can Fail People with Diabetes*, American Diabetes Association and Georgetown University Health Policy Institute, February 8, 2005, http://web.diabetes.org/Advocacy/healthresearchreport0505.pdf.

9 J. M. McWilliams, A. M. Zaslavsky, E. Meara, and J. Z. Ayanian, "Impact of Medicare Coverage on Basic Clinical Services for Previously Uninsured Adults," *Journal of American Medical Association* 290 (2003): 757–64; J. Z. Ayanian, J. S. Weissman, E. C. Schneider, J. A. Ginsburg, and A. M. Zaslavsky, "Unmet Health Needs of Uninsured Adults in the United States," *JAMA* 284 (2000): 2061–69; D. W. Baker, J. J. Sudano, J. M. Albert, E. A. Borawski, and A. Dor, "A Lack of Health Insurance and Decline in Overall Health in Late Middle Age," *New England Journal of Medicine* 345 (2001): 1106–12; J. M. McWilliams, A. M. Zaslavsky, E. Meara, and J. Z. Ayanian, "Health Insurance Coverage and Mortality among the Near-Elderly," *Health Affairs* 23, no. 4 (2004): 223–33.

10 J. M. McWilliams, E. Meara, A. M. Zaslavsky, and J. Z. Ayanian, "Use of Health Services by Previously Uninsured Medicare Beneficiaries," *New England Journal of Medicine* 357 (July 12, 2007): 143–53.

11 The survey is the Current Population Survey (CPS), which is conducted every month and surveys more than fifty thousand households across the country. The CPS is the source for monthly estimates of the unemployed numbers. Every month (except December), additional questions are asked about specific topics, and since 1980, questions about health insurance have been included in the March supplemental survey. The questions related to health insurance coverage ask about specific types of health insurance (e.g., employer-sponsored coverage, Medicare, Medicaid, self-purchased policies), and only people who answer "no" to every question are considered uninsured. This means that someone who may have been uninsured for part of the previous year but had employer-sponsored coverage in the other months is not counted as uninsured.

12 People can be uninsured for quite different lengths of time. Some people lose health insurance when they lose a job and then gain it again if they get a job with coverage—this could take only a month or several months. Other people may be uninsured for years because they are in jobs that do not have group health insurance as a benefit and they cannot afford to purchase their own individual policies. Studies of spells without health insurance show that about half of them last no more than six or seven months—but another quarter of all spells go on for a year or more; see K. Swartz, J. Marcotte, and T. D. McBride, "Spells without Health Insurance: The Distribution of Durations when Left-Censored Spells Are Included," *Inquiry* 30, no. 1 (2003): 77–83. Several studies using surveys that followed people for two or four years show that between 30 and 38 percent of the population younger than sixty-five were uninsured for at least a month, and 9 to 12 percent were always uninsured; see P. F. Short, D. R. Graefe, and C. Schoen, "Churn, Churn, Churn: How Instability of Health Insurance Shapes America's Uninsured Problem," *Issue Brief* (New York: Commonwealth Fund, November 2003); P. F. Short and D. R. Graefe, "Battery-Powered Health Insurance? Stability in Coverage of the Uninsured," *Health Affairs* 22, no. 6 (2003): 244–55; K. Klein, S. Glied, and D. Ferry, "Entrances and Exits: Health Insurance Churning, 1998–2000," Issue Brief (New York: Commonwealth Fund, September 23, 2005). These numbers bracket the estimate that almost 18 percent of the population under sixty-five were uninsured in 2006 and illustrate how the dynamics of health insurance coverage affect the estimates of how many people are uninsured. If we restrict our focus to people who are long-term uninsured, we estimate a smaller number of uninsured; and if we include anyone who has gone at least a month without coverage over a year's time, we estimate a larger number.

13 The Appendix contains tables showing the age, education, and family income

distributions of the uninsured in 1979 and 2006, and the simple probability of being uninsured in 1979 and 2006 for different cohorts (by age, education, and family income).

14 Households are comprised of single individuals as well as married-couple families and related families. As a result, 56 percent of all individuals in 2006 were middle class—they were either individuals or in families with incomes greater than the median household income.

15 In 1979, 10.8 million children were uninsured; they accounted for 17 percent of all children and 39 percent of the uninsured population under age sixty-five.

16 The Omnibus Budget Reconciliation Act of 1987 expanded Medicaid eligibility such that now states must cover all children ages six to eighteen with family incomes below the poverty level, and all children under age six with family incomes below 133 percent of the poverty level. States have the option of covering children with incomes up to 185 percent of the poverty level.

17 See, for example, Kaiser Commission on Medicaid and the Uninsured, "Health Coverage of Children: The Role of Medicaid and SCHIP," *Key Facts,* September 2007, http://www.kff.org/medicaid/children.cfm; T. M. Selden, J. L. Hudson, and J. S. Banthin, "Tracking Changes in Eligibility and Coverage Among Children, 1996–2002," *Health Affairs* 23, no. 5 (2004): 39–50.

18 D. Cutler and J. Gruber, "Does Public Insurance Crowd Out Private Insurance?" *Quarterly Journal of Economics* 111, no. 2 (1996): 391–430; J. Gruber and K. Simon, "Crowd-Out Ten Years Later: Have Recent Public Insurance Expansions Crowded Out Private Health Insurance?" National Bureau of Economic Research, *Working Paper No. 12858* (2007).

19 A. Sommers, S. Zuckerman, L. Dubay, and G. Kenney, "Substitution of SCHIP for Private Coverage: Results from a 2002 Evaluation in Ten States," *Health Affairs* 26, no. 2 (2007): 529–37; G. Kenney and A. Cook, "Coverage Patterns among SCHIP-Eligible Children and Their Parents," The Urban Institute, February 2007, http://www.urban.org/url.cfm?ID=311420.

20 S. A. Camarota, "Immigrants in the United States, 2007: A Profile of America's Foreign-Born Population," *Background Report* (Washington, DC: Center for Immigration Studies, November 2007).

21 C. Schoen, M. M. Doty, S. R. Collins, and A. L. Holmgren, "Insured But Not Protected: How Many Adults Are Underinsured?" *Health Affairs* Web Exclusive w5 (June 14, 2005): 289–302, http://content.healthaffairs.org/cgi/reprint/hlthaff.w5.289v1. See also earlier estimates of the underinsured population: P. J. Farley, "Who Are the Underinsured?" *Milbank Quarterly* 63, no. 3 (1985): 476–503, and

P. F. Short and J. S. Banthin, "New Estimates of the Underinsured Younger than 65," *JAMA* 274, no. 16 (1995): 1302–6.

22 The percentage of the nonelderly population covered by ESI held steady in the mid-1990s (at 64.6 percent on average) and then increased in the second half of the 1990s to a high of 68.4 percent in 2000 (P. Fronstin, "Sources of Health Insurance and Characteristics of the Uninsured: Analysis of the March 2007 Current Population Survey," *Issue Brief No. 310* (Washington, DC: Employee Benefit Research Institute, October 2007). The decline since 2000 is the longest since the CPS began to ask questions about health insurance coverage in 1980.

23 G. Claxton, I. Gil, B. Finder, B. DiJulio, S. Hawkins, J. Pickreign, H. Whitmore, and J. Gabel, *Employer Health Benefits: 2006 Annual Survey* (Menlo Park, CA: Henry J. Kaiser Family Foundation; Chicago, IL: Health Research and Educational Trust, 2006).

24 K. Swartz, *Reinsuring Health: Why More Middle-Class People Are Uninsured and What Government Can Do* (New York: Russell Sage Foundation, 2006).

25 G. Claxton, J. Gabel, B. DiJulio, J. Pickreign, H. Whitmore, B. Finder, P. Jacobs, and S. Hawkins, "Health Benefits in 2007: Premium Increases Fall to an Eight-Year Low, While Offer Rates and Enrollment Remain Steady," *Health Affairs* 26, no. 5 (2007): 1407–16.

26 Ibid.

27 Ibid.

28 Agency for Healthcare Research and Quality, Center for Financing, Access and Cost Trends, Medical Expenditure Panel Survey, 2003, Insurance Component, Table I.A.2, http://info.ahrq.gov.

29 J. Haas and K. Swartz, "The Relative Importance of Worker, Firm, and Market Characteristics for Racial/Ethnic Disparities in Employer-Sponsored Health Insurance," *Inquiry* 44, no. 3 (2007): 280–302; P. J. Cunningham, *Choosing To Be Uninsured: Determinants and Consequences of the Decision to Decline Employer-Sponsored Health Insurance* (Washington, DC: Center for Studying Health System Change, 1999); P. F. Cooper and B. S. Schone, "More Offers, Fewer Takers for Employment-Based Health Insurance: 1987 and 1996," *Health Affairs* 16, no. 6 (1997): 142–49.

30 The payroll taxes are primarily for Social Security and Medicare, which together equal 7.65 percent of earnings (up to $97,500 in 2007 for Social Security but with no maximum for Medicare). Employers also do not pay these payroll taxes on what they pay for health insurance premiums (or premium equivalents if the employers self-insure their workers' health care costs). In addition, workers do

not pay income taxes on the amount of money that the employer pays for the premium; this particularly benefits higher income workers who face higher marginal tax rates.

31 L. Burman, "Taking a Check Up on the Nation's Health Care Tax Policy: A Prognosis," Statement before the U.S. Senate Committee on Finance, March 8, 2006.

32 Tax Policy Center, The Urban Institute and Brookings Institution, Table T07-0054: Current Law Tax Benefits for Health Insurance, Distribution of Subsidies by Cash Income Class, Nondependent Tax Units with Head or Spouse Under 65, February 6, 2007, http://www.taxpolicycenter.org/numbers/displayatab.cfm?DocID=1457.

33 See http://www.whitehouse.gov/stateoftheunion/2007/initiatives/healthcare.html. For an analysis of the proposed standard deduction for health insurance, see L. Burman, J. Furman, G. Leiserson, and R. Williams, *The President's Proposed Standard Deduction for Health Insurance: An Evaluation*, Urban Institute and Brookings Institution Tax Policy Center, February 14, 2007, http://www.taxpolicycenter.org/UploadedPDF/411423_Presidents_Standard_Deduction.pdf. Many people believe the Bush administration's proposal would encourage employers to stop offering ESI. Workers would then face higher premiums than they pay now because the advantages of group purchasing by employers, especially large employers, would no longer exist.

34 I. Lurie and B. Heim, "Do Increased Premium Subsidies Affect How Much Health Insurance Is Purchased? Evidence from the Self-Employed," paper presented at the Association for Public Policy Analysis and Management Annual Meeting, November 2007.

35 For example, in Massachusetts, before the health insurance reform legislation was passed in 2006, about 900,000 people were covered by small-group policies and only about 45,000 people were covered by individual market policies. Massachusetts has a labor market that provides strong incentives for small firms to offer ESI so the relative shares of people covered by the two markets is probably more extreme there than in other states.

36 The commission in Massachusetts charged with evaluating the likely effects of merging the small-group and individual markets estimated that premiums for people who had been covered by small-group policies would go up between 1 and 1.5 percent and premiums for people who had been purchasing coverage in the individual market would be reduced by 14 percent.

37 Swartz, *Reinsuring Health*.

38 All of the HMOs in the state must participate in Healthy New York (HNY) — just as they must participate in the state's standard individual (self-pay) insurance market.

The benefits package for HNY is leaner than that in the individual market, and people in HNY are subject to somewhat higher cost-sharing expenses. The reinsurance funds come from the state's Tobacco Settlement Funds.

39 This is similar to the logic behind requiring people to pay taxes for Social Security, Medicare, and general government services.

40 See http://www.healthpass.com; and S. N. Rosenberg, "New York's HealthPass Purchasing Alliance: Making Coverage Easier for Small Businesses," Commonwealth Fund Report No. 662, September 2003, http://www.commonwealthfund .org/usr_doc/rosenberg_nyhealthpass_662.pdf?section=4039.

41 The federal tax code allows employers to create Section 125 plans that permit employees to place some of their income in an account to pay for certain benefits, including health insurance. The money the employee puts in the plan is not subject to federal or state taxes, including Social Security and Medicare payroll taxes — so a person can pay the premiums for health insurance with pretax income if the employer creates a Section 125 account for that purpose.

42 If a person chooses a plan with a deductible, the nominal premium will be lower. The highest deductible in 2006 was 500 euros (or about $650 at the exchange rate in 2006) per person. See the Royal Netherlands Government, Ministry of Health, Welfare and Sport, "The New Care System in the Netherlands," May 2006; http:// www.minvws.nl/en/folders/z/2006/the-new-health-insurance-system-in-three-languages.asp.

43 Technically, the individuals pay the 6.5 percent tax on their income up to 30,150 euros but employers are required to reimburse this amount to their employees.

44 D. M. Cutler and M. McClellan, "Is Technological Change Worth It?" *Health Affairs* 20, no. 5 (2001): 12–29.

45 K. Swartz, "Revising Employers' Role in Sponsoring and Financing Health Insurance," in *A Future of Good Jobs? America's Challenge in the Global Economy*, ed. T. Bartik and S. Houseman (Kalamazoo, MI: W. E. Upjohn Institute, 2008).

46 J. Hadley and J. Holahan, "How Much Medical Care Do the Uninsured Use, and Who Pays for It?" *Health Affairs* Web Exclusive w3 (February 12, 2003): 66–81.

47 J. Hadley and J. Holahan, "Covering The Uninsured: How Much Would It Cost?" *Health Affairs* Web Exclusive w3 (June 4, 2003): 250–65.

CHAPTER THREE

Get Sick, Go Broke

DEBORAH THORNE & ELIZABETH WARREN

No family wants to file for bankruptcy. To do so is an unmistakable sign of personal failure.[1] It is an indelible mark that the person filing will remember long after the creditors have moved on and the court records have been archived. For a family facing bankruptcy in the aftermath of a medical problem, the pill is especially bitter. Unfortunately, about half of all families filing for bankruptcy do so as the result of a serious medical problem.[2]

Moreover, bankruptcy files reveal that America's health insurance system offers no guarantees that those with medical problems will be spared. Fully three-quarters of people filing medical bankruptcies reported that they had insurance at the onset of the illness or accident that ultimately tied into their financial failure. For these families, the concept of "coverage" fell far below the reassuring protection that they believed they had. The bankruptcy data expose the weakness of a health insurance system that is riddled with co-payments, benefit caps, excluded illnesses, and uncovered expenses.

For too many hard-working middle-class families, a single bad diagnosis or a modest accident can mean financial ruin. Even a relatively routine event such as an appendectomy or the long-term care of diabetes can devastate a family's budget. Taken together, the work of many researchers strongly suggests that America is facing a crisis in health care. Since

2000, an estimated five million families have filed for bankruptcy in the aftermath of serious medical problems.[3] But those five million families are only the visible tip of a very large iceberg. For every family filing for bankruptcy, economic experts estimate that another sixteen families are in serious enough financial trouble that they would benefit from bankruptcy—if only they were willing to file.[4] The current health care system is bankrupting hard-working, play-by-the-rules American families.

In this chapter, we will examine the diversity and frequency of medical bankruptcies. We will explore data showing the vulnerability of families with health insurance, and the various ways in which families try to pay their medical expenses. We will also discuss changes to our nation's health care system that could reduce the financial impact of a serious medical problem.

COLLECTING THE DATA

Data for the findings presented in this chapter come from the 2001 Consumer Bankruptcy Project.[5] We collected self-administered questionnaires and court records for 1,250 bankrupt households from five bankruptcy districts around the United States.[6] We also conducted follow-up telephone interviews with 602 of the 1,250 respondents. Combined, the three instruments provided an opportunity to determine which respondents experienced medical bankruptcies.

In general, the families that file for bankruptcy are not concentrated among the chronically poor. Instead, they are people who have been to college, gotten decent jobs, bought homes, and started families.[7] Most are wage earners, although about one is seven has run a small business.[8] In other words, when measured by the most enduring criteria, the families in bankruptcy are our neighbors and friends, a sample of middle-class and working-class America. Right up until the bills piled up or the time lost from work left them unable to cover basic expenses, these families never dreamed they would end up in a bankruptcy court.

DEFINING MEDICAL BANKRUPTCY

In 1978, bankruptcy laws were modernized in part to reflect a changing consumer economy. From 1980 until 2004, filings generally followed a strong upward trend, increasing from 250,000 filings to 1.5 million in twenty-five years. In 2005, Congress amended the bankruptcy laws, leaving a six-month window before the harsher new provisions went into effect. Predictably, filings jumped to over two million in 2005, then dropped back to 600,000 in 2006, before beginning to climb back up in 2007.[9] Filings are currently on track to break one million again in 2008.[10]

Our data suggest that many of these bankruptcies were medical bankruptcies. For example, about 46 percent of respondents who completed the telephone interview self-identified a specific illness or injury among their explanations for filing bankruptcy.[11] From C-sections to cancer, car accidents to complications from diabetes, families themselves identified the illnesses and accidents, births and deaths that contributed to their financial collapse.

For many other families, it was unpaid time lost from work that hit them the hardest and led to their bankruptcies. About one in five debtors (21 percent) indicated that they had lost at least two weeks' income because of a medical problem. In some cases, the primary wage earner was ill. In others, a child, spouse, or elderly relative required care and the wage earner had to miss work to provide it. Either way, the loss of income for medical reasons constituted a hard financial blow for families.

Other medical bankruptcies occurred when families mortgaged (or re-mortgaged) their homes to get the cash needed to pay medical debts. The numbers were modest, only about 2 percent of the total sample, which translated to about 4 percent of the homeowners surveyed. The impact on family finances, however, was often quite serious. When a family re-mortgages the home or adds a second mortgage, the debt must be paid off in full, plus any penalties and interest. If the family cannot make those payments, bankruptcy will offer little help and the family will lose its home.[12]

Many of those who mortgaged their homes or lost time from work identified themselves as filing for bankruptcy at least in part because of medical problems. When these families are combined with the self-identifiers, the percentage of medical-related bankruptcies increases to 56 percent (see Figure 3.1).

Other responses from filers produced inferences of medical-related financial problems. About a quarter (26 percent) of the debtors reported having medical bills in excess of $1,000 in the two years before filing

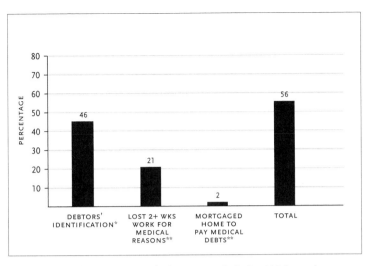

Figure 3.1   Medical bankruptcies: medical reasons, medical-related job loss and mortgages to pay medical debts, by percent [Source: 2001 Consumer Bankruptcy Project (*phone interview and self-administered questionnaire combined; N=602) (**self-administered questionnaire only; N=1250)]

that were not covered by insurance. Out-of-pocket medical expenses of $1,000 may seem too small to suggest that a medical problem contributed to a family's financial demise, but for families with modest incomes, the burden is considerable. Among the families filing for bankruptcy, median annual income was about $25,000, and even at the eightieth percentile, income was only about $40,000. Of course, $1,000 is only the threshold number. The telephone surveys completed by a subset of the sample revealed medical debts at much higher amounts: respondents reported average out-of-pocket medical expenses of $11,854.[13]

About 2 percent of the sample identified alcohol and drug problems as reasons for filing. For parents who explained that they had bankrupted themselves putting their teenaged children through substance abuse rehabilitation programs, this reason would be an appropriate inclusion. For others for whom the story is one of drunken profligacy, characterization as a medical bankruptcy might seem inappropriate. Similarly, some researchers would want to include the 1 percent of the sample who identified a family member's gambling problem as a medical reason for filing, recognizing that some families get left behind financially when a spouse or parent goes on a gambling binge, loses the house, and leaves

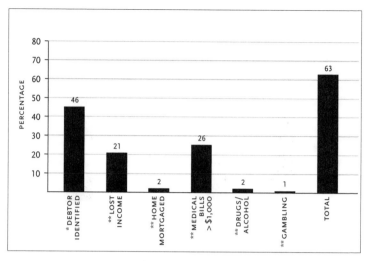

Figure 3.2   Medical-related bankruptcy, all sources, by percent

[Source: 2001 Consumer Bankruptcy Project (*phone interview and self-administered questionnaire combined; N=602)

(**self-administered questionnaire only; N=1250)]

everyone deep in debt. Others would see gambling as a moral failure or a simple risk calculation, unrelated to any medical condition.

When the definition of a medical bankruptcy is expanded to include $1,000 or more of out-of-pocket medical bills in the two years prior to bankruptcy, alcohol/drug abuse, and gambling, the percentage of medical bankruptcies climbs to 63 percent (see Figure 3.2).

If the families we studied in the 2001 Consumer Bankruptcy Project are representative of bankruptcy filers nationwide, this would mean that an estimated 668,000 to 915,000 families filed for bankruptcy in 2001 at least in part due to medical-related financial distress.[14] These numbers pale in comparison with the debtors who have similar problems but have managed to somehow avoid bankruptcy.[15] But they show that by any analysis, the economic stress on families struggling with medical problems is unmistakable.

WHICH MEDICAL EXPENSES CAUSE THE MOST TROUBLE?

We know that families filing medical bankruptcy struggle with "medical" bills, but what exactly does that mean? Depending on the type of medical

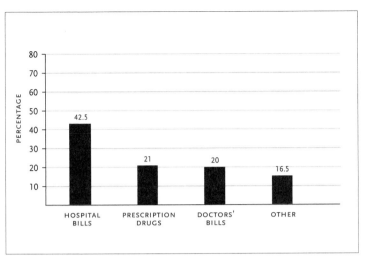

Figure 3.3   Medical bills of bankrupt families, by percent

[Source: 2001 Consumer Bankruptcy Project (phone survey; N=196)]

bill, there are varying implications for the family and the health of the members. For example, hospital bills may result in a lawsuit or lien against the home. An inability to pay doctor bills may mean that wages are garnished or that a particular doctor may refuse to see the patient again. Struggling to pay for prescription drugs may translate into family members taking partial dosages or skipping them altogether—or to loading up on credit card debt.

About 42.5 percent of medically bankrupt families identified hospital bills as their single biggest expense.[16] But the role of hospital bills must be kept in perspective. The fact that hospital bills are one of many different kinds of significant medical expenses for families of modest means should not be surprising. Consumers' out-of-pocket payments to hospitals are only a tiny fraction of overall out-of-pocket medical payments in the United States.[17]

This is reflected in the fact that nearly 60 percent of families reported that their biggest medical expenses were something other than a hospital bill. As Figure 3.3 illustrates,[18] about one fifth (21 percent) identified prescription drugs as their biggest expense.[19] Another fifth (20 percent) identified doctor bills as their biggest expense.[20] Studies in the medical literature have emphasized the role of nonhospital medical expenses when they evaluate cost-related underuse of health services and drugs.[21] In one recent study, the overwhelming majority of older Americans reported no out-of-pocket expenses for hospital or nursing home care, but most had other kinds of out-of-pocket medical expenses.[22]

INCOME AND MEDICAL DEBTS

The complexity of medical bankruptcy is reflected by the fact that medical-related indebtedness often results from something *other than* direct medical bills.[23] For example, among those who had identified a medical reason for filing in the telephone survey sample, four out of ten (40.1 percent) said that medical debt was *not a factor at all* in their decision to file.[24] Half (50.8 percent) said that prescription drug costs were not a factor at all. Instead, for many families, medical bankruptcies resulted from a loss of income. As noted earlier, about one in five debtors (21 percent) indicated that they had lost at least two weeks' income because of a medical problem.[25] And among those who indicated in the telephone survey they had filed for medical reasons, eight of ten (80.2 percent) reported that income loss due to health problems contributed "very much" or "somewhat" to their bankruptcies.[26]

Complicating the role of income loss is the fact that the bankruptcy filers often were not themselves the ill or injured person. Instead, they lost income while taking care of sick relatives.[27] Of the medical bankruptcy filers who had lost substantial time from work as a result of a medical problem, more than half (52.8 percent) did so to care for someone else.[28] In 13.3 percent of the medical bankruptcy cases involved in the follow-up telephone survey, primary earners were caring for a sick child.[29] The filers tell stories of premature births and chronically ill or disabled children with persistent and demanding care needs. Among those in the sample were parents who reported missing months of work when a child with spinal bifida required repeated operations, when a baby was born with heart defects, or when an infant with sickle cell anemia needed special care. One parent faced substantial work disruptions because of an autistic child, and yet another lost income to deal with an epileptic child. A child with severe bipolar and anxiety disorder required twenty-four hour monitoring, leading first to significant leaves of absence and eventually to job loss for the child's mother. After being told by doctors that their son with kidney problems would die, one set of parents moved the entire family to a different state with hopes of better treatment and a different prognosis.

Other filers reported losing income to care for spouses, aging parents, or other relatives. One man reported caring for his wife while she battled lung cancer, while another went back to work only after his wife had three operations in six months and finally was able to walk down the hallway of their home without his help. An adult daughter struggled to help with her mother's medical bills not covered by Medicare and eventually took unpaid family leave so she could take her mother for medical treatments.[30] Adult children temporarily or permanently moved in with parents to help them cope with the effects of Alzheimer's disease or terminal illnesses. One man cared for an uncle with cancer while trying to raise a toddler grandson and assist his son with college.

The statistics and stories show the often-ignored income side of the health care debates. The financial impact of a serious medical problem can reverberate through a family in many ways.

WHEN HEALTH INSURANCE IS NOT ENOUGH

Most current health policy debates revolve around how to provide health insurance for those who do not have it. The assumption is that health insurance will shield families from the most severe financial consequences of a health care problem. But the bankruptcy data suggest something quite different. Insurance does not always prevent illnesses and injuries from spiraling into financial catastrophes. Participants in the study explained that the combination of co-pays, insurance limits, and coverage exclusions left even those with comprehensive health insurance responsible for thousands of dollars in expenses. Moreover, during the course of a serious illness, some families saw their health insurance canceled or coverage denied, leaving them without protection at the exact moment when they were most vulnerable.

According to our data, many people filing for medical bankruptcy actually had health insurance, at least at the onset of the medical problems that contributed to their bankruptcies. Almost seven out of ten (67.4 percent) medical filers said all family members had insurance at the time of the filing.[31] The family member with the medical problem was covered at even higher rates; more than three-quarters of the families in bankruptcy reported that the ill or injured person had insurance at the time the person fell ill.[32] Despite these high rates of insurance coverage, medical debt caused extreme financial difficulty for these families.

These data are consistent with several other empirical studies. For example, a study of individuals who filed for bankruptcy in 1999 reported a high rate of insurance coverage among bankruptcy filers who indicated that a medical problem contributed to their financial troubles.[33] National and local studies by groups such as the Commonwealth Fund, the Center for Studying Health System Change, the Kaiser Family Foundation, and the Access Project have observed significant financial vulnerability and medical indebtedness even among the insured.[34]

These findings come as no surprise to hospital executives and other commentators who observe that co-pays and deductibles among insured patients can be a significant part of a hospital's bad debt.[35] But they come as a harsh blow to insured families as they discover that no matter how hard pressed they may be, many hospitals treat co-pays, deductibles, and the like as ineligible for charity care.[36]

The bankruptcy data also serve as a reminder that "insured" and "uninsured" are dynamic categories. Among the families listing themselves as medically bankrupt, one-third of those with private coverage at the onset of their medical problems reported that they lost coverage at some point during the course of their treatment.[37]

The revelations regarding the high rates of insurance among the families declaring medical bankruptcy provoked a harsh response from the insurance industry. Anxious to refute our findings that three-quarters of the medically bankrupt in the United States had health insurance and the resulting spotlight on inadequate coverage and insurance cancellation practices, the industry sponsored an attack on the study.[38] The researchers, Dranove and Millenson, collected no new data, nor did they reanalyze our data. Instead, they redefined "medical bankruptcy" to exclude those who were overwhelmed by the costs of prescription medications, those who mortgaged their homes to pay medical bills, and those who lost more than two weeks of unpaid time from work. We disagree with their attempts to redefine what qualifies as a medical bankruptcy and stand firmly by our criteria and conclusion that hundreds of thousands of families with health insurance are filing bankruptcy each year in the aftermath of serious medical problems.

The insured are surely luckier than their uninsured counterparts, but these data show that they remain vulnerable. Those with health insurance find their way into bankruptcy—even into medical bankruptcy—in numbers that match the uninsured.[39]

THE CREDIT TRAP

As a result of inadequate health insurance coverage, families often have little choice but to convert their medical bills into ordinary consumer credit. About three in ten (29.3 percent) families identifying medical bankruptcies reported using credit cards for medical expenses.[40] For some, the amount of medical debt carried on credit cards was modest, while for others, the numbers were truly staggering. For example, after insurance did not cover an emergency baby delivery, one new parent charged the entire $17,000 bill to a credit card, starting a chain of financial problems that ended in complete collapse. Another family used credit cards to finance monthly thousands of dollars of medications for a child with non-Hodgkins lymphoma because insurance would pay for blood transfusions but not drugs. One filer in our study used credit cards to buy medical supplies associated with a loved one's cancer treatments. These findings suggest that a substantial portion of the debts listed in bankruptcy may appear as ordinary purchases on credit cards when, in fact, they represent the cost of medical services.

Some families go into debt even more deeply to try to pay medical bills. Recall that about 4 percent of homeowners in the written questionnaire sample mortgaged their homes to pay medical bills.[41] Among homeowners who had taken second or third mortgages on their homes in the months before bankruptcy, fully 15 percent had taken this step to finance their medical expenses. By the time they file for bankruptcy, these families may owe nothing directly to a health care provider, but they will be paying this medical debt (and the accumulated interest) for years. If they cannot pay, these families face losing their homes, all in an effort to pay their medical bills.

Bankruptcy filers are not alone in their use of consumer credit for medical expenses. Nationally representative studies have found families using personal loans, credit cards, and mortgages to finance medical bills.[42] According to Visa, patients charged $19.5 billion in health care services to

Visa cards in 2001, which was made possible by the fact that most medical practices now accept credit cards.[43] And a study by Dēmos revealed that 29 percent of low- and middle-income households with credit card balances reported that medical expenses contributed to their current debt loads.[44]

In addition to the use of general purpose credit for medical care, some medical providers have forged informal (and unpublicized) relationships with lenders to provide credit to their patients to finance their care.[45] Many lenders offer medical-specific credit products with providers such as the Citi® Health Card,[46] CareCredit (a division of GE Retail Sales Finance),[47] AccessOne,[48] MedCash,[49] PXpert,[50] the King Thomason Group TotalCare Medical Accounts Receivable Credit Card Program,[51] the HELPcard,[52] MediCredit,[53] and HelpEZ.[54] As a result, the Federal Trade Commission has noted the existence of a "well-established market" for medical-specific loans.[55]

Families with pressing financial problems have turned to consumer debt in their efforts to honor their medical bills. Rising out of families' medical misfortune is an industry eager to provide high-priced credit. The story of health care in the United States is increasingly a story of indebtedness.

PAYING FOR HEALTH CARE:
A PRIMARY CONCERN FOR ALL AMERICANS

The American health care system is impressive for all of its scientific advances. But the system also exacts a high price from many insured and uninsured American families. The troubling signs of a broken health care system have become obvious to millions of families. In 2007, half of all Americans said they were worried about paying medical costs if they became seriously ill or had an accident.[56] Our findings suggest that these concerns are justified.

We approach the health care debates from a single perspective: maintaining the financial stability of families confronting illness or injury. The most obvious solution would be universal single-payer health care. This would allow people to get the care they need—without risking bankruptcy to pay for it. No more credit card debt at 29.9 percent interest to pay for drugs; no more second mortgages to pay for a hospital admission; no more dealing with debt collectors who garnish wages and threaten to put liens on homes. Single-payer care would also free families from dependence on an employer's plan and make certain that everyone is covered, whether or not they are employed. We recognize that there are cost-containment issues and the ever-present specter of rationing medical care. But from the perspective of family finances, this is the most obvious and workable solution.

If universal, single-payer health insurance is politically unacceptable, then another option would be to guarantee all Americans access to *affordable and adequate* health insurance that cannot be terminated or made more costly if a family member is ill or injured. Moreover, health insurance should not be tied to employment. As these data show, when the employed family member is ill or injured, or must care for a loved one, employment-based health insurance can be lost. The economic consequences of this are often catastrophic. It may be commendable for employers to provide affordable and adequate health insurance, but they should not be in the position to determine who is covered and whether that coverage meets basic family needs.[57]

Health care innovations that are designed to change the delivery of health care and contain costs could also be structured to stave off the heavy financial impact of a serious medical problem. Although most such efforts are aimed at less expensive treatments, such as preventive care and routine treatments delivered through low-cost clinics, reforms that make prescription drugs and rehabilitation therapy available at low or no cost would relieve the financial burdens of a significant number of families.

We also note that medical problems can quickly evolve into income problems. The bankruptcy data show that people lose significant time from work, not only for their own medical problems, but also for the illnesses and accidents that befall their children, spouses, and elderly relatives. Policies that provide paid leave for care providers would go a long way toward alleviating these difficulties—working Americans should not have to choose between earning an income and caring for a seriously ill or dying loved one. Another approach would be to expand health care delivery, providing more assistance for caring. In-home care could help families maintain their financial footing during a relative's recuperation or a family member's decline. The idea of shared care—with family members and outside workers sharing the work of caring—would not only be less expensive than complete residential care, it would also be a better, more loving solution for many families.

Finally, we sound a note of warning. Since 1980, the movement in law has been toward deregulation of consumer financial products. For those buying iPods and sneakers on their credit cards, the consequences can be serious when interest rates escalate and penalty fees kick in. But for those who are ill, the deregulation trend in consumer lending is genuinely frightening. A new industry is taking root to profit from the financing of health care. The medical-credit industry is as unregulated as other parts of consumer credit, but the purchaser has even fewer options and less ability to weigh the ordinary consequences of buying on credit versus delaying a purchase. Delaying repairs to the car is one thing; delaying treatments for a potentially terminal illness is another. Policymakers should act immediately to put meaningful regulations on the extension of medical credit to stop health care providers from shifting a medical debt problem to an even more serious consumer credit problem. The bottom line is clear: People should not be gouged for getting sick.

The financial fallout of even a modest medical problem can bankrupt all but the wealthiest families. The bankruptcy data show that millions of families are tumbling over the economic edge for reasons that are beyond their control. Medical bankruptcy data are sparse, but earlier studies suggest that medical bankruptcies increased twenty-five-fold from 1980 to 2001.[58] The bankruptcy amendments of 2005 raised the costs of bankruptcy and reduced the number of people who were eligible for relief, but there is no reason to believe that the underlying problems that prompted more than five million medical bankruptcy filings between 2001 and 2007 have diminished.

The bankruptcy data are a visible aspect of a serious national problem. If the costs of medical care are not borne collectively, millions more families will find that even if they can recover physically from an accident or illness, the lives they have worked so hard to build will be lost to them forever.

NOTES

1   Deborah Thorne and Leon Anderson, "Managing the Stigma of Personal Bankruptcy," *Sociological Focus* 39, no. 2 (2006): 77–97.

2   David U. Himmelstein, Deborah Thorne, Elizabeth Warren, and Steffie Woolhan-
    dler, "Illness and Injury as Contributors to Bankruptcy," *Health Affairs* Web Exclu-
    sive w5 (February 2, 2005): 69, http://content.healthaffairs.org/cgi/reprint/hlthaff
    .w5.63vi. Also see Melissa Jacoby and Elizabeth Warren, "Beyond Hospital Misbe-
    havior: An Alternative Account of Medical-Related Financial Distress," *Northwest-
    ern University Law Review* 535 (2006): 100.

3   From 2000 until the first half of 2007, 10.5 million households filed for bank-
    ruptcy. Administrative Office of the United States Courts, "Bankruptcy Statistics,"
    available at: http://www.uscourts.gov/bnkrpctystats/bankruptcystats.htm. If about
    half of these families filed medical bankruptcies, as the data suggest, then about
    five million families made the trip to the bankruptcy court in the aftermath of a
    serious medical problem.

4   Michelle J. White, "Why It Pays To File Bankruptcy: A Critical Look at the Incen-
    tives Under the U.S. Personal Bankruptcy Law and a Proposal for Change," *Univer-
    sity of Chicago Law Review* 65, no. 3 (1998): 702. About 17 percent of all households
    would have benefited financially from filing bankruptcy—at a time when about 1
    percent of households were filing.

5   For a thorough discussion of our research methods, see the Appendix to Elizabeth
    Warren and Amelia Tyagi, *The Two Income Trap: Why Middle Class Mothers and
    Fathers Are Going Broke* (New York: Basic Books, 2003).

6   A total of 1,250 questionnaires, 250 from each district, were collected. At the back
    of each questionnaire, respondents were asked if, for $50 each, they would com-
    plete up to three follow-up telephone interviews.

7   Elizabeth Warren, "Financial Collapse and Class Status: Who Goes Bankrupt?"
    Osgoode Hall Law Journal 41, no. 1 (2003): 115. Of the sample, 57.2 percent had been
    to college, 56.3 percent had jobs in the upper 80 percent of occupational prestige
    scores, 58.3 percent were homeowners, and 91.8 percent had one or more of these
    indicia of class status.

8   Robert Lawless and Elizabeth Warren, "The Myth of the Disappearing Business
    Bankruptcy," *California Law Review* 93, no. 3 (2005): 745.

9   Administrative Office of the United States Courts, "Bankruptcy Statistics," avail-
    able at: http://www.uscourts.gov/bnkrpctystats/bankruptcystats.htm.

10 Robert M. Lawless, "U.S. Bankruptcy Filings Up from One Year Ago But Leveling
    Off," *Credit Slips,* http://www.creditslips.org (accessed December 12, 2007). Every
    quarter since the reforms the numbers of filings have climbed. In 2007, bank-
    ruptcy filings exceeded 800,000. If the current trend continues, consumer filings
    for 2008 will surpass one million.

11 Note that the total number of respondents drops from the questionnaire data alone (1,250) because the response rate on the follow-up telephone surveys was about half (N=602) of all the families that completed questionnaires. This means that any data that combine the paper questionnaires and telephone surveys can use only the smaller N from the telephone surveys. Because the "reasons" information is drawn from two sources instead of one, it is both different and more complete than the data first reported in Himmelstein et al., "Illness and Injury."

12 In a limited class of cases, a second or third mortgage may be discharged, but only if the earlier mortgages have already exceeded the value of the home.

13 Consumer Bankruptcy Project, N=331 (core plus supplemental homeowner telephone survey sample, unweighted).

14 To estimate the number of families that will be affected, we use the data on bankruptcies from the Administrative Office of the United States ("AO") courts. We follow the AO classification of cases into "business" and "nonbusiness," using the "nonbusiness" classification as a proxy for the number of households filing for bankruptcy. In other work, the AO methods for distinguishing between business and nonbusiness cases have been criticized because the count of "nonbusiness bankruptcies" includes approximately 300,000 self-employed debtors, many of whose small businesses have failed; see Robert Lawless and Elizabeth Warren, "The Myth." In addition, the way in which the AO data are reported has changed over time, and this makes it difficult to evaluate trends in business and nonbusiness filing rates from the mid-1980s. For the purposes of this work, however, the difficulties in distinguishing nonbusiness filers from self-employed filers is less important. Whether they are wage earners or entrepreneurs, the nonbusiness bankruptcies represent a household in financial trouble, and this is the appropriate unit of analysis here.

15 See, for example, USA Today/Kaiser Family Foundation/Harvard School of Public Health, *Health Care Costs Survey,* Summary and Chartpack, chart 3 (August 2005), which reported that only a small percentage of the sample who indicated medical-related financial distress filed bankruptcy, http://www.kff.org/newsmedia/upload/7371.pdf); Amanda E. Dawsey and Lawrence M. Ausubel, *Informal Bankruptcy,* February 2002, http://www.ausubel.com; Michelle J. White, "Personal Bankruptcy Filing under the 1978 Bankruptcy Code: An Economic Analysis," *Indiana Law Journal* 63 (Fall 1987): 50 (finding that more households would benefit from bankruptcy than actually file). The Cambridge Consumer Credit Index (press release, February 7, 2005), based on a poll of over eight hundred adults, reported that "83 percent of Americans say that debts they have incurred because of medical or dental procedures are burdensome enough to prevent them from buying large ticket items,"

http://www.cambridgeconsumerindex.com/index.asp?content=press_release.

16 Consumer Bankruptcy Project, N=331 (core plus supplemental homeowner telephone survey sample, unweighted). See Himmelstein et al., "Illness and Injury," 69. Because these data came from the telephone survey instead of the written questionnaire, the N is smaller (see note 11). The question about medical expenses was asked only of the subset of debtors taking the telephone survey who identified medical problems.

17 U.S. Census Bureau, *Statistical Abstract of the United States: 2004–2005*, 95, tables no. 120–121 (reporting $14.7 billion in out-of-pocket consumer payments to hospitals, and $212.5 billion overall out-of-pocket payments in 2002; payments to hospitals were less than those to physicians and clinical services [$34.2 billion], prescription drugs [$48.6 billion], and nursing home care [$25.9 billion]).

18 Consumer Bankruptcy Project, N=196. For those with continuous coverage who identified significant medical debt (N=83), we asked about the single greatest expense. The combination of the two groups comprises Figure 3.3. The category "other" includes insurance premiums, medical equipment, nursing home care, in-home care, and other unspecified expenses.

19 See ibid. Among those filers eligible for Medicare and with psychiatric disorders, prescription drugs were the biggest expense for nearly all of them. Also see Kenneth M. Langa et al., "Out-of-Pocket Health-Care Expenditures among Older Americans with Cancer," *Value in Health* 7, no. 2 (March 2004): 191 (a nationally representative study of older Americans finding that prescription drugs were the main source of increased out-of-pocket expenses among people undergoing cancer treatment). Whether or not the elderly will be aided by the Medicare prescription drug bill (Medicare Prescription Drug, Improvement, and Modernization Act of 2003, Pub. L. No. 108–173, 117 Stat. 2469 [December 8, 2003]), those with trouble affording medications are not necessarily Medicare-eligible; see, e.g., J. Kennedy and C. Erb, "Prescription Noncompliance Due to Cost among Adults with Disabilities in the United States," *American Journal of Public Health* 92, no. 7 (July 2002): 1123 (in the sample, 27 percent of those with problems paying for drugs were eligible for Medicare).

20 Himmelstein et al., "Illness and Injury," 69. See also Jeffrey Prottas, "Costs, Charges, and Medical Debt: What is the Real Goal?," *American Heart Hospitals* 3, no. 1 (2005): 43 (observing that complaints about hospital collection practices may be applicable to other types of medical providers).

21 See, e.g., Jeffrey J. Ellis et al., "Suboptimal Statin Adherence and Discontinuation in Primary and Secondary Prevention Populations," *General Internal Medicine* 19

(2004): 638; A. D. Federman, "Don't Ask, Don't Tell: The Status of Doctor-Patient Communication about Health Care Costs," *Archives of Internal Medicine* 164, no. 16 (September 13, 2004): 1723; Dana P. Goldman et al., "Pharmacy Benefits and the Use of Drugs by the Chronically Ill," *JAMA* 291, no. 19 (May 19, 2004): 2344; H. A. Huskamp et al., "The Effect of Incentive-Based Formularies on Prescription Drug Utilization and Spending," *New England Journal of Medicine* 349, no. 23 (2003): 2224; Kennedy and Erb, "Prescription Noncompliance"; John D. Piette et al., "Problems Paying Out-of-Pocket Medication Costs Among Older Adults With Diabetes," *Diabetes Care* 27 (2004): 384; John D. Piette et al., "Cost-Related Medication Underuse: Do Patients with Chronic Illnesses Tell Their Doctors?," *Archives of Internal Medicine* 164 (2004): 1749; D. Safran et al., "Prescription Drug Coverage and Seniors: How Well are States Closing the Gap?," *Health Affairs* Web Exclusive w2 (July 31, 2002): 253, http://content.healthaffairs.org/cgi/reprint/hlthaff.w2.253v1; M. A. Steinman et al., "Self-Restriction of Medications Due to Cost in Seniors without Prescription Coverage," *General Internal Medicine* 16, no. 2 (December 2001): 793–99; R. Tamblyn et al., "Adverse Events Associated With Prescription Drug Cost-Sharing Among Poor and Elderly Person," *JAMA* 285, no. 4 (January 24, 2001): 421; and, summarizing recent studies, Rebecca Voelker, "Cost Is an Adverse Drug Effect, Patients Cut Corners and Risk Health," *JAMA* 292, no. 18 (November 10, 2004): 2201.

22 See, e.g., Langa et al., "Out-of-Pocket Health-Care Expenditures," 190.

23 More than a quarter of all filers in the 2001 written questionnaire sample identified illness or injury as a reason for filing, whether or not they owed large medical debts; see Himmelstein et al., "Illness and Injury," 67, Exhibit 2 (N=1771). See generally, Melissa Jacoby, Teresa Sullivan, and Elizabeth Warren, "Rethinking the Debates over Health Care Financing: Evidence from the Bankruptcy Courts," *New York University Law Review* 76, no. 2 (2001): 388 (54.9 percent of those who said illness or injury was a reason for filing for bankruptcy did not identify a current debt to a medical provider).

24 Consumer Bankruptcy Project, N=331 (core plus supplemental homeowner telephone survey sample, unweighted).

25 Consumer Bankruptcy Project, N=1,250. The rate is nearly identical (21.3 percent) if the homeowner sample is added and weighted into the analysis as well. See Himmelstein et al., "Illness and Injury," 67, Exhibit 2.

26 Jacoby and Warren, "Beyond Hospital Misbehavior," 535. The filers' narrative accounts, even if not representative, also illustrate the range of circumstances in which income loss follows both longer term and acute problems. For example,

open-heart surgery and its aftermath led to loss of temporary work and a resulting loss of income for one filer. Others told interviewers they had missed too much work due to chronic illness or hospitalizations and either could not work out an arrangement with employers or were advised by doctors to take different types of jobs. Doctors ordered bed rest for pregnant women who had been in car accidents or who had developed gestational diabetes; one consumed all her allotted family leave before the baby was born, and soon after was fired. A number of others explained that they had difficulty receiving their workers' compensation benefits or were receiving benefits at levels far below their prior incomes.

27 See generally B. F. Hughes et al., "Pediatric Femur Fractures: Effects of Spica Cast Treatment on Family and Community," *Journal of Pediatric Orthopedics* 15, no. 4 (July–August 1995): 457 (discussing costs of casting for femur fractures, including average of three weeks of lost work for parent in families with two working parents); and Carol E. Smith et al., "Efficiency of Families Managing Home Health Care," *Annals of Operations Research* 73, no. 1 (1997): 157.

28 See Himmelstein et al., "Illness and Injury," 69.

29 Ibid.

30 See Chizuko Wakabayashi and Katharine Donato, "Does Caregiving Increase Poverty among Women in Later Life? Evidence from the Health and Retirement Survey," *Journal of Health and Social Behavior* 47 (September 2006): 258–74 (reporting that when women are caregivers earlier in their lives, they are more likely to experience poverty when they are older).

31 Consumer Bankruptcy Project, N=1,771 (core plus homeowner written questionnaire sample, weighted). The figure for nonmedical filers was 65.5 percent, but the difference was not statistically significant.

32 More than eight of ten (82.7 percent) of the ill or injured person(s) were insured at the time they were interviewed (core plus homeowner telephone survey sample, unweighted, measured by people instead of cases); Consumer Bankruptcy Project, N=329. The percentage calculated by cases rather than people results in a similar figure, 82.83 percent; Consumer Bankruptcy Project, N=331.

33 See Jacoby et al., "Rethinking the Debates," 399–404 (finding about 80 percent of petitioners insured at time of filing, including about 80 percent of medical-related filers).

34 See, e.g., USA Today et al., *Health Care Cost Survey,* chart 1 (reporting that 61 percent of those having trouble paying medical bills were insured); Cathy Schoen et al., "Insured But Not Protected: How Many Adults are Underinsured?," *Health Affairs* Web Exclusive w5 (June 14, 2005): 289, http://content.healthaffairs.org/cgi/content/abstract/hlthaff.w5.289v1 (finding 12.3 percent of nonelderly adults are

underinsured); Sara R. Collins et al., "The Affordability Crisis in U.S. Health Care: Findings from the Commonwealth Fund Biennial Health Insurance Survey," http://www.commonwealthfund.org/usr_doc/collins_biennial2003_723.pdf?section=4039 (noting that two of five adults had medical bill problems or accrued medical debt even though 62 percent had insurance); Jessica H. May and Peter J. Cunningham, "Tough Trade-Offs: Medical Bills, Family Finances, and Access to Care," Center for Studying Health System Change (2004), http://www.hschange.org/CONTENT/689/689.pdf (finding about forty-three million people have medical debt problems even though about two-thirds have insurance); National Public Radio, Kaiser Family Foundation, and Harvard University Kennedy School of Government, *Survey on Health Care* (2002), http://www.kff.org/insurance/20020605a-index.cfm (stating that over one fifth of families reported medical debt problems, including 15 percent of those with insurance). See also Deborah Gurewich et al., "Medical Debt and Consumer Credit Counseling Services," *Journal of Health Care for the Poor and Underserved* 15, no. 3 (2004) 340 (noting that about 75 percent of those with medical illnesses contributing to financial problems in Florida credit counseling sample reported having insurance at illness onset, and over half of insured reported having large medical debt); Carol Pryor and Deborah Gurewich, "Getting Care but Paying the Price: How Medical Debt Leaves Many in Massachusetts Facing Tough Choices" (2004), http://www.accessproject.org/downloads/MAreport.pdf (reporting that over 40 percent in Massachusetts community health center user sample had medical debt problems, including almost 30 percent of those with insurance); Kaiser Family Foundation, Kaiser Commission on Medicaid and the Uninsured, "Challenges and Trade-Offs in Low-Income Family Budgets: Implications for Health Coverage" (2004), http://www.kff.org/medicaid/4147.cfm (finding insured low-income families with medical debt).

35 See, e.g., Richard Haugh and Dagmara Scalise, "A Surge in Bad Debt: High Co-Pays and Deductibles Mean More Patients Can't Pay Hospital Bills in Full," *Hospital and Health Networks* 77, no. 12 (December 2003): 14; Sharona Hoffman, "Unmanaged Care: Towards Moral Fairness in Health Care Coverage," *Indiana Law Journal* 78 (2003): 661; William D. White, "Market Forces, Competitive Strategies, and Health Care Regulation," *University of Illinois Law Review* no. 1 (2004): 162 ("[T]he net result of these cost sharing strategies is to expose employees to large out-of-pocket outlays in the event of serious illness"); Patrick Reilly, "Indigent-Care Spending Low," *Modern Healthcare* 34, no. 8 (February 23, 2004): 7 (stating that increased cost-sharing is contributing to hospital bad debt).

36 See, e.g., "A Review of Hospital Billing and Collections Practices: Hearing Before the Subcommittee on Oversight and Investigations of the House Committee on

Energy and Commerce," 108th Cong. (June 24, 2004): 283 (making clear that Ascension Health's charity care policy is inapplicable to co-payments and deductibles of insured payments and providers of medical savings accounts).

37 N=331 (core plus supplemental homeowner telephone survey sample, weighted). The group that lost coverage amounts to 19 percent of the telephone survey medical sample. For the debtors' reasons for losing coverage, see Himmelstein et al., "Illness and Injury," w5: 67, exhibit 3. Gaps in coverage seem to correlate with greater out-of-pocket costs. In the written questionnaire sample, medical filers had a higher rate of reporting a gap in insurance than nonmedical filers. Over a third (38.4 percent) of medical bankruptcy filers in the written questionnaire sample reported at least a one-month lapse in insurance coverage for anyone in the household. When evaluating this finding, however, it is important to keep in mind that some of those who reported this gap may be uninsured at the time of filing. Among the telephone survey medical sample, ill or injured people with private coverage at illness onset, but who later lost it, reported an average of $18,005 in out-of-pocket costs since onset as compared to those without any gap ($9,898). See Himmelstein et al., "Illness and Injury," 69–70, exhibit 5.

38 David Dranove and Michael L. Millenson, "Medical Bankruptcy: Myth versus Fact," *Health Affairs* 25, no. 2 (2006): 74–83.

39 See Prottas, "Costs, Charges, and Medical Debt": "[The] uninsured suffer the most, but the insured poor also carry a heavy burden of debt, and the problem is far from unusual among the middle class.... Focusing on the uninsured is a reasonable way to start, but it is clearly inadequate" (41); "Insurance failure is clearly contributing to the medical debt problem, perhaps on a scale comparable to the un-insurance problem" (42).

40 Consumer Bankruptcy Project, N=331 (core plus supplemental homeowner telephone survey sample, unweighted). This figure jumps to more than half (51.4 percent) if the filers with medical problems who charged basic necessities that may relate to health or general well-being are included.

41 See Himmelstein et al., "Illness and Injury," 67, exhibit 2.

42 See, e.g., Collins et al., "The Affordability Crisis," 18 (one fifth of those with medical bill problems or medical debts charged large debts to credit cards or used home mortgages); Piette et al., "Problems Paying Out-of-Pocket Medication Costs," 387 (14 percent of patients in sample, and 23 percent of those without drug insurance coverage, increased credit card debt to be able to afford prescription drugs); Ha T. Tu, "Rising Health Costs, Medical Debt and Chronic Conditions," Center for Studying Health System Change, *Issue Brief No. 88* (September 2004): 3, http://www

.hschange.org/CONTENT/706/706pdf (50 percent of working-age adults with chronic conditions whose families had problems paying medical bills in past year had to borrow money to pay); Glenn B. Canner et al., "Recent Developments In Home Equity Lending," *Federal Reserve Bulletin* 84 (1998): 248, table 8 (increase in borrowers indicating medical expenses as use for home equity loans). Other studies have reported the use of consumer credit in categories that have included medical debt. See, e.g., Peter J. Brady et al., "The Effects of Recent Mortgage Refinancing," *Federal Reserve Bulletin* (July 2000): 446 (39 percent of 1998 and early 1999 refinancings used for consumer expenditures, which includes medical expenses); HUD-Treasury Task Force on Predatory Lending, "Curbing Predatory Home Mortgage Lending," June 2000, p. 31, http://www.treas.gov/press/releases/reports/treasrpt .pdf (citing a National Home Equity Mortgage Association survey finding that 30 percent of subprime home equity loans were used for covering medical, educational, and other expenses, as compared to 25 percent for home improvement and 45 percent for debt consolidation); Javier Silva, "A House of Cards: Refinancing the American Dream," *Dēmos, Borrowing to Make Ends Meet Briefing Paper #3* (January 2005), http://www.demos-usa.org/pubs/AHouseofCards.pdf (discussing Federal Reserve System Flow of Funds data from 2001–2002 showing that 25 percent of home equity funds were used for consumer expenditures, including medical expenses). See generally Heather C. McGhee and Tamara Draut, "Retiring in the Red; The Growth of Debt Among Older Americans," *Dēmos, Borrowing to Make Ends Meet Briefing Paper #1* (January 2004), p. 6, http://www.demos-usa.org/pubs/Retiring_2ed.pdf (discussing role of medical costs in increased credit card debt among older Americans).

43 See Julie A. Jacob, "Credit to Your Practice: Letting Patients Pay With Plastic," *American Medical News,* July 29, 2002, http://www.ama-assn.org/amednews/ 2002/07/29/bisa0729.htm.

44 Cindy Zeldin and Mark Rukavina, "Borrowing to Stay Healthy: How Credit Card Debt is Related to Medical Expenses," Dēmos and the Access Project, 2007, http:// www.accessproject.org/adobe/borrowing-to-stay-healthy.pdf.

45 See generally Robert W. Seifert, "The Demand Side of Financial Exploitation: The Case of Medical Debt," *Housing Policy Debate* 15, no. 3 (2004): 795. See also Johnson v. Rutherford Hosp. and Murfreesboro Bank & Trust Co., 13 B.R. 185 (Bankr. M.D. Tenn. 1981) (hospital arranged for credit).

46 Citibank Health Card Program, http://www.citibank.com/us/cards/cardserv/ healthcrd/cons_benefits.htm.

47 See http://www.carecredit.com; Tyler Chin, "In the Cards: Getting Paid with Plastic; Innovations in the Credit and Debit Card Industry Are Giving Physicians New

Options for Collecting Bills," *American Medical News*, January 12, 2004, http://www
.ama-assn.org/amednews/2005/01/12/bisa0112.htm (GE Sales Finance declined
to discuss in detail but said it was targeting high dollar specialty practices).

48 See http://www.accessonemedcard.com; Mike Stobbe, "Credit Card Agency Cuts Hospitals' Losses," *Charlotte Observer,* July 11, 2003 (discussing AccessOne program).

49 See Michael Unger, "Just What the Doctor Ordered: Schein's One-Stop Service
Ranges from Equipment to Personal Finance," *Newsday,* December 30, 1996, C7.

50 See news release, "PracticeXpert Launches PXpert Medical Credit Card Program,"
September 4, 2003, http://www.primenewswire.com/newsroom/news.htm/?d=
4608 (acquiring delinquent accounts from physician, transferring balance to
credit card); Chin, "In the Cards" (PracticeXpert program will be targeting patients
with poor credit histories).

51 See news release, "King Thomason Group Enters into Agreement with Medical
Capital Corporation to Market KTG's TotalCare Medical Accounts Receivable Credit
Card Program," April 23, 2004, www.kgth.com/main/totalrecovery.htm (citing 95
approval rate for private pay patients). KTG also offers a structured payment plan
as an alternative to credit cards.

52 http://www.helpcard.com/consumer/helpisprovided.html.

53 This credit product is used by patients of the Inova Health System, to be distinguished from the financier of cosmetic surgery with the same name.

54 http://www.healthEZ.com (encouraging employers to offer as supplement to health
plans); Larry Werner, "War Stories about Start-up Funding Leave 'Em Laughing,"
Minneapolis Star Tribune, July 2, 2003, 1D.

55 See Federal Trade Commission Commentary on Fair and Accurate Credit Transac-
tions Act of 2003, Medical Information Rulemaking (May 27, 2004).

56 Bill Novelli, "Where We Stand," *AARP Bulletin* 31 (July–August 2007) (citing a 2007
Gallup Survey of 1,008 adults). More than a quarter — 28 percent — describe themselves as "very worried" and another 21 percent say they are moderately worried.

57 See Brigitte C. Madrian, "Employment-Based Health Insurance and Job Mobility:
Is There Evidence of Job-Lock?" *Quarterly Journal of Economics* 109, no. 1 (1994):
27–51 (suggesting a 25 percent reduction in job mobility when health insurance
was tied to employment). See also Jonathan Gruber and Brigitte C. Madrian,
"Health Insurance and Job Mobility: The Effects of Public Policy on Job-Lock,"
Industrial and Labor Relations Review 48, no. 1 (October 1994): 86–102 (reporting
that when health insurance benefits are continued, employees are more likely to
change jobs, thus, job-lock is less likely to occur).

58 Himmelstein et al., "Illness and Injury," 5–71.

CHAPTER FOUR

Just How Good *Is* American Medical Care?

ELIZABETH A. MCGLYNN, DAVID MELTZER,

& JACOB S. HACKER

For decades, American medical care has been portrayed as the best in the world—a utopia of high-tech treatments, cutting-edge research, and expeditious and effective interventions. In this still-dominant view, the problems in U.S. health care concern cost and access, not the quality of care that Americans receive. In recent years, however, this glossy image has come under increasing scrutiny.[1] A large and growing body of research—some of it longstanding but much of it emerging in the last decade—has carefully examined the question "Just how good is American medical care?" The answer, it turns out, is "sometimes excellent, but much more uneven and unexceptional than many once thought."

To be certain, the best American medical care is extremely good. Yet there is a substantial gap in the United States between what is known to work and what is being done for patients. American adults, for example, receive just half of recommended care for the leading causes of death and disability, and the proportion is similarly low for children.[2] At the same time, despite spending much more per person on health care than any other nation, the United States does not consistently outperform other rich countries on quality measures.[3]

In short, American medical care has plenty of room for improvement. Yet upgrading medical quality is not, as many policymakers today seem to believe, merely a matter of expanding coverage. Broader coverage is good for many reasons, but it is no guarantee that insured Americans will receive the care they need. Nor is quality improvement a sure ticket to lower costs — another common misconception. Quality sometimes saves money; at other times, it costs more. By the same token, many ideas for cost control — from lower provider payments to greater individual cost sharing — have blunt effects on quality, reducing necessary and unnecessary interventions alike.[4] If the quality of American medical care is to be improved, it will need to be the explicit focus of policy changes, not a hoped-for byproduct.

Indeed, what recent evidence shows most strongly is that quality of care is less about the level of resources devoted, or even the form of medical financing, than it is about how care is actually delivered in the places where patients are treated. Improving our knowledge of how the structure of delivery affects both medical quality and health outcomes — and how that knowledge can be applied to make Americans healthier and American medical care better—should be a top priority in the coming debate over national health reform.

WHAT DO AMERICANS THINK ABOUT HEALTH CARE QUALITY?

As other chapters in this volume discuss in more depth, health care is a top concern of Americans. Much of the concern understandably centers on issues of affordability and coverage — the two pillars of health security. For example, two-thirds of persons identifying themselves as Republicans and almost 90 percent of Democrats said in a survey published in January 2008 that they were dissatisfied with the costs of health care in this country.[5] That a substantial minority of Americans do not have health insurance was viewed as a somewhat or very serious problem by 83 percent of Republicans and 100 percent of Democrats. Not surprisingly, cost and access have been major areas of national political discussion in recent years. Health care quality, by contrast, has not generated the same sort of intense debate.

One potential explanation for the relatively small amount of attention to health care quality is that Americans just do not worry about quality. Yet we know this is not the case: When asked if they were satisfied with the quality of care on this country, 40 percent of Republicans and

78 percent of Democrats said no.[6] This dissatisfaction does not seem to be primarily a reflection of current personal experience, since only 10 percent of Republicans and 23 percent of Democrats said they were dissatisfied with their *own* care. However, it also does not appear to reflect only selfless concern about the care received by others. Instead, a major source of Americans' worries about medical quality appears to be the perceived *insecurity* of the (perceived to be relatively high quality) care they now receive. Although the vast majority of Americans say their current care is of high quality, most do not expect it to stay that way: In this recent survey, more than half of Republicans and 68 percent of Democrats said they are worried about the worsening of the quality of health care services they receive.

One reason for this concern may be the fear of losing health coverage and, in turn, receiving lower quality care. Fully 43 percent of Republicans and 59 percent of Democrats in the same survey expressed at least some worry about losing coverage. A plausible interpretation of these results is that Americans largely equate access to care with quality: "If I can just get in the door, everything will be okay and if my policy pays for all the important things I need if I get really sick, then I will get those interventions."

Indeed, when asked to name the most important health care issues in deciding their vote, 61 percent of Republicans and 73 percent of Democrats said that either cost or lack of universal coverage was most important to them, while only 22 percent of Republicans and 18 percent of Democrats said that improving quality of care and reducing medical errors were most important. This suggests that health care quality is an important concern for some Americans, but that this may reflect more general concerns about continuing access to care rather than quality of care for patients with insurance.

WHAT IS QUALITY CARE?

Americans are not alone in finding it hard to distinguish between costs, access, and quality. Although virtually everyone can agree that the quality of medical care is a distinct dimension of health system performance, defining "quality" turns out to be notoriously difficult. In an influential 1990 report, the Institute of Medicine (IOM) defined the quality of medical care as the "degree to which health services for individuals and populations increase the likelihood of desired health outcomes and are consistent with current professional knowledge."[7] In practical terms, poor quality can mean too much care, too little care, or the wrong care. More recently, the IOM has acknowledged that quality is multidimensional, and has identified six domains that together constitute health system quality: effectiveness, safety, timeliness, patient-centeredness, equity, and efficiency: "Good quality means providing patients with appropriate services in a technically competent manner, with good communication, shared decision making, and cultural sensitivity."[8] Within these domains, quality can be measured in terms of whether the conditions exist to deliver good care (structure), whether the right clinical processes were provided (technical process), whether care was delivered in a manner that was acceptable to the patient (interpersonal process), and whether the best possible results were achieved (outcomes).[9]

In what follows, we focus mostly on the effectiveness of care using technical process measures. From this perspective, quality of care is the degree to which effective methods of prevention, screening, diagnosis, treatment, and follow-up are actually delivered by health care providers. This means that quality assessment requires knowing what methods of care are effective in improving patient health. Once these methods are known, then it is possible to examine how often and when providers of care actually use them appropriately. The advantage of such process indicators is that they reflect the way providers think about what they do and the way the underlying science is organized. As such, technical process measures represent an appropriate approach to accountability. Other potential measures of quality, such as general health outcomes or clinician qualifications, are less useful in this regard. General health outcomes reflect other influences on health besides what providers do, whereas structural measures like clinician qualifications may not be good predictors of what is actually done. That said, we bring into our discussion other domains and types of measures when they can reasonably be seen as useful for system accountability.

THE QUALITY OF CARE FOR AMERICAN ADULTS

Until recently, the degree to which health care in the United States was consistent with basic quality standards remained largely unknown.

Although studies had documented serious quality deficits, they provided limited perspective. Most had assessed a single condition, a small number of indicators of quality, persons with a single type of insurance coverage, or persons receiving care in a small geographic area.[10] Meanwhile, the few national studies were limited to specific segments of the population, focused on a limited set of topics, or assessed health outcomes without a link to specific processes involved in care. This information gap contributed to a persistent belief that quality was not a serious national problem.

In the 1990s, one of us (McGlynn), working with a team of researchers, sought to fill this gap by examining the extent to which the recommended processes of medical care—one critical dimension of quality—were delivered to a representative sample of the U.S. population for a broad spectrum of conditions in twelve metropolitan areas (Boston; Cleveland; Greenville, South Carolina; Indianapolis; Lansing, Michigan; Little Rock, Arkansas; Miami; Newark, New Jersey; Orange County, California; Phoenix, Arizona; Seattle; and Syracuse, New York). The indicators of quality used in the study were derived from RAND's Quality Assessment Tools system, a comprehensive, clinically based system for assessing the quality of care for children and adults.[11] The indicators cover a wide range of clinical areas and all four *functions* of medicine: screening, diagnosis, treatment, and follow-up. The indicators also cover a variety of *modes* of providing care, such as history, physical examination, laboratory study, medication, and other interventions and contacts.

Overall, this comprehensive study found that participants received just over half (54.9 percent) of recommended care. This level of performance was similar in the areas of preventive care, acute care, and care for chronic conditions. The level of performance did not vary much by medical function, ranging from 52.2 percent for screening to 58.5 percent for follow-up care. There was greater variation, however, among modes. Care requiring an encounter or other intervention (e.g., the annual visit recommended for patients with hypertension) had the highest rates of adherence (73.4 percent), whereas processes involving counseling or education (e.g., advising smokers with chronic obstructive pulmonary disease to quit smoking) had the lowest rates of adherence (18.3 percent).

As noted already, poor quality care may involve too much care or too little. The greatest problem turned out to be undertreatment

(46.3 percent of recommended care was not delivered), rather than overtreatment (11.3 percent of care that was not recommended and was potentially harmful was delivered). The quality of care also varied greatly by the conditions that patients had. For example, people with senile cataracts received 78.7 percent of recommended care, yet persons with alcohol dependence received just 10.5 percent of recommended care.

Worryingly, the quality of care was poor even in clinical domains where timely and effective treatment is well established and leads to substantial and proven health gains. Only 24 percent of participants in the study who had diabetes, for instance, received three or more glycosylated hemoglobin tests over a two-year period. This routine monitoring is essential to the assessment of the effectiveness of treatment, to ensuring appropriate responses to poor glycemic control, and to the identification of complications of the disease at an early stage so that serious consequences may be prevented. Similarly, while 68 percent of the recommended care for coronary artery disease was received, only 45 percent of persons presenting with a myocardial infarction received beta-blockers, which reduce the risk of death by 13 percent during the first week of treatment and by 23 percent over the long term.

The same was true with preventive care: Actions that are known to save lives were routinely not taken. Among elderly participants, only 64 percent had received or been offered a pneumococcal vaccine; nearly ten thousand deaths from pneumonia could be prevented annually by appropriate vaccinations. About 38 percent of participants had been screened for colorectal cancer; annual fecal occult-blood tests could prevent about ninety-six hundred deaths annually.

Finally, much room for quality improvement existed in all of the communities studied. Even in the community with the highest score, less than 60 percent of effective care was delivered on average.[12] Although some communities performed better than others in selected clinical domains, in general there was little variation among these metropolitan areas. The relative rankings of the communities changed depending on the aspect of care under examination. But no community performed markedly better than others overall, and all showed serious gaps between what we know should be done and what was done.

In short, the deficits in the quality of care represent a national problem—one that has to be seen as posing a serious threat to the health and well-being of the American public.

THE QUALITY OF CARE FOR AMERICAN CHILDREN

Over the past twenty years, as other chapters in this volume have discussed, there has been a major expansion of public health insurance for low-income children—first, with the extension of Medicaid to a larger share of the poor, and then with the creation and growth of the State Children's Health Insurance Program. Yet expanding access is only part of the challenge of ensuring that children receive necessary services. If there are major deficits in the delivery of care to children, then expanding coverage alone will not be enough.

Unfortunately, most research on the quality of care has focused on adults rather than children. Moreover, past studies of the quality of care provided to children have many shortcomings, such as limited quality measures; reliance on self-reported data from parents, patients, or providers; and exclusive attention to Medicaid enrollees or a single geographic area. Building on the study of the quality of care for adults just described, a parallel study examined the quality of care delivered to children. It began by using established national guidelines and the medical literature to develop indicators of quality for the continuum of care functions—including screening, diagnosis, treatment, and follow-up—for the most common childhood health care needs. A review of medical records from all individual and institutional providers seen over a two-year period provided the information needed to determine whether each child was eligible for the care represented by each indicator and whether the required care had been received.

The bottom-line of the study was very similar to what was found with adults. On average, children received just 46.5 percent of recommended care. They received 67.6 percent of the indicated care for acute medical problems, 53.4 percent of the indicated care for chronic medical conditions, and only 40.7 percent of the indicated preventive care. Adherence rates for the continuum of care functions ranged from 37.8 percent of indicated screening processes to 65.9 percent of indicated treatment processes. Care processes requiring that the provider prescribe a specific medication had the highest rates of adherence (81.0 percent), and those requiring laboratory or imaging services had the lowest rates of adherence (36.3 percent). As with adults, the rates of adherence were lower for indicators characterized by underuse of services (42.4 percent) than for those characterized by overuse (73.1 percent) or misuse (90.2 percent).

These results suggest that many children are at risk of adverse health outcomes because of quality deficits. For example, only 44 percent of children with asthma who were noted to be using beta-2 agonists at least three times per day had a prescription for an anti-inflammatory medication recorded in the chart. Children with persistent asthma who are treated with inhaled anti-inflammatory drugs have fewer asthma-related symptoms and improved pulmonary function,[13] are hospitalized less frequently,[14] and have lower asthma-related mortality[15] than those who are not treated. Similarly, immunizations are effective in protecting children against a variety of serious childhood diseases; yet only 49.8 percent of children who reached two years of age during the study period were fully immunized, according to their records.

The list of potential problems goes on. Urine cultures were obtained for just 16.2 percent of children three to thirty-six months of age who presented with fever of unknown origin and who were thought to be at high risk for sepsis. The reported prevalence of urinary tract infection is high (4 to 5 percent) among children two months to two years of age who have fever without an identified source of infection on the basis of the history and physical examination. Early diagnosis of urinary tract infection might lead to earlier identification of high-grade vesicoureteral reflux, allowing for the prevention of recurrent infections, worsening renal damage, and chronic renal failure.[16]

No less worrisome, only 41.5 percent of eligible adolescent girls in the current study had charts showing evidence of laboratory orders for tests for chlamydia trachomatis or of the results of such testing. Screening for chlamydia is important, because 75 percent of such infections are asymptomatic, and it is reported that 40 percent of untreated women and adolescents will have pelvic inflammatory disease. Of that 40 percent of women, 20 percent will have infertility due to tubal factors and 9 percent will have life-threatening complications during pregnancy.[17] Broad-based screening, early detection, and treatment have decreased the incidence of pelvic inflammatory disease associated with chlamydia in adolescent girls by 60 percent, lowering rates of hospitalization and complications.[18]

In sum, deficits in the quality of care for children turn out to be similar in magnitude to those previously reported for adults. Although ensuring that children have health coverage is a valuable goal, it will not, by itself, eliminate these serious gaps in the quality of care.

U.S. HEALTH CARE QUALITY IN CROSS-NATIONAL PERSPECTIVE

If American children and adults receive only about half of indicated care, are there other nations that do consistently better? The answer is no. There are nations that do better on some important quality indicators than we do, but there is no universally high-performing system. However, other nations are investing heavily in electronic medical records and measures to increase health system accountability. These investments could greatly improve quality — and perhaps leave the United States behind.

Part of the difficulty in assessing comparative medical quality is that no country routinely and comprehensively measures quality. In a recent comprehensive analysis sponsored by the Commonwealth Fund, for example, a team of researchers started with about one thousand quality measures collected in one or more countries and ended up with just twenty-one indicators for five nations (and only sixteen that could be applied across the board in all five). The measures themselves are, by the researchers' own admission, an opportunistic set that does not give a comprehensive picture of quality in any of these countries.

Nonetheless, taking these limits as given, the twenty-one indicators strongly suggest that when it comes to quality, all good things do not go together. No country was the top or bottom performer in all the twenty-one areas for which comparative data were available. In the United States, breast cancer survival rates were relatively high, as were cervical cancer screening rates. At the same time, asthma mortality rates were increasing in the United States but decreasing in the other countries, and transplant survival rates were low. The researchers concluded: "While the United States often performs relatively well for this set of indicators, it is difficult to conclude that it is getting good value for its medical care dollar from these data.... Earlier studies have shown the

United States to be in the bottom quartile of population health indicators such as life expectancy and infant mortality. Our results also fail to reveal what the extra spending has bought."[19]

Other recent analyses have suggested an even less favorable picture of American performance. The Commonwealth Fund has supported a number of additional large-scale studies of U.S. health care in cross-national perspective, relying primarily on surveys of physicians and patients in a half dozen or so affluent nations. When it comes to quality, the first study suggests, the United States performs better than it does on other dimensions (such as "access," "equity," and "efficiency"). In particular, Americans are relatively more likely to receive "treatments that, according to evidence-based guidelines, are effective and appropriate for a given condition—in other words, *the right care*."[20] But the United States does less well, according to the survey evidence, in chronic care management and the provision of safe, coordinated, and patient-centered care—areas in which other countries have been investing increasing resources.

To be sure, Americans are generally confident they will receive the latest medical technology (only the Dutch are markedly more so), and they experience comparatively short waits for elective surgery. Yet American adults often report waits for primary care, find it difficult to get care after hours, and end up seeking care from emergency rooms—problems in primary care infrastructure that the United States shares with Canada. And, of course, compared with citizens of other nations, many more Americans say they have postponed or delayed care because of the cost.

If the growing body of comparative quality research does not support the claim that there is a "best system" (much less that the United States is that system), it does begin to suggest where quality efforts will need to focus—and why quality improvement will need to be its own agenda in health care reform, not simply an afterthought.

WHAT MATTERS LESS THAN COMMONLY THOUGHT

If quality is a problem even in nations with some form of national health insurance, then it is safe to conclude that access does not ensure quality. (On the other hand, there is no evidence that national health insurance inevitably means poor quality care either.) This is a conclusion that policymakers sometimes find hard to believe, but it is wholly consistent with a wealth of research. There is no evidence, for example, that clinical quality in the United States is consistently better or worse in fee-for-service than in health maintenance organizations (HMOs).[21] The appropriateness of many surgical procedures is similar in the United States, Canada, and the United Kingdom—three vastly different systems, one of which leaves a third of its nonelderly population uninsured at some point every two years.

Nor is the amount spent on health care systematically related to quality, at least among rich nations with high spending. Health care as a proportion of gross domestic product varies from 8.3 percent in the United Kingdom to 16 percent in the United States. It is true that the United Kingdom has not performed well on some key quality indicators—which might suggest that spending is the issue. And yet, the UK actually excels in other areas. Meanwhile, the United States does not consistently outperform other nations in the domain of quality, despite spending more than twice as much per capita as the United Kingdom and fully 50 percent more than the next highest-spending nation, Switzerland.

Thus, there is good reason to believe that controlling spending is not inherently inimical to maintaining quality. Better management of chronic conditions in outpatient settings can prevent costly hospitalizations. Influenza and pneumonia vaccines reduce hospitalizations as well as prevent deaths. Improved management of depression has been associated with improved health and increased rates of employment. Still, not all improvements in quality will reduce costs, especially given the prevalence of underuse. Put bluntly, we simply do not know the net effects on health spending of comprehensive strategies to improve quality.

What we do know is that spending restraint by itself has blunt effects on quality. For example, studies of efforts in New Hampshire to reduce prescription drug costs found that these efforts reduced the use of both necessary and unnecessary medications. Similarly, eliminating payment for ineffective medications in New Jersey was associated with an overall increase in the number of prescriptions and resulted in both desirable and undesirable clinical substitutions. Cost sharing reduced overall spending on antibiotics, but appropriate and inappropriate uses were reduced at the same rate.

Fortunately, thanks to recent research and real-world practice, we now understand much better what can be done to improve quality. And perhaps the most telling lessons come from a surprising American success story—the transformation of the Veterans Health Administration (VHA), the largest health delivery system in the United States, into one of the best integrated medical models in the world.

A SURPRISING STORY OF HIGH-QUALITY CARE

When problems came to light in the Walter Reed Medical Center in Maryland in 2007, thanks to a Pulitzer Prize-winning series in the *Washington Post,* many commentators assumed that the scandalously bad care received by veterans there was just one more example of poor quality services for the nation's returning soldiers. Movies like *Born on the Fourth of July* have portrayed veterans' care as grossly substandard—an image that, at one time, contained a good deal of truth. But in fact Walter Reed is not part of the VHA; it is run by the Defense Department, not the Department of Veterans Affairs. And the VHA is anything but substandard. Indeed, it may well be, as one recent book puts it, "the best care anywhere."[25]

No single statistic better illustrates this remarkably good performance than the share of VHA system participants who receive recommended care. In the rest of the American health system, as we have already reported, adults and children receive only about half of the care that they should. The figure in the VHA is just over two-thirds.[26]

How does the VHA do it? Beginning in the early 1990s, VHA leadership instituted both a sophisticated electronic medical record system and a quality measurement approach that holds regional managers accountable for several processes in preventive care and in the management of common chronic conditions. Other changes included a system-wide commitment to quality improvement principles and a partnership between researchers and managers for quality improvement.

The VHA is the largest health care system to have implemented these quality-related system changes, and the reforms have worked: The VHA has substantially better quality of care than found in the rest of American health care. Although present research does not indicate exactly why VHA care is so much better, it appears that the VHA's promulgation of specific performance measures and emphasis on accountability are at the heart of the system's success. The use of computerized reminders and electronic records; the emphasis on standing orders, improved interprovider communication, facility performance profiling, leveraging of academic affiliations, and accountability of regional managers for performance; and the creation of a more coordinated delivery system—in tandem, all these reforms have allowed VHA medical care to create and uphold very high standards of quality.

AN AGENDA FOR QUALITY IMPROVEMENT

What the surprising story of the VHA suggests is that for quality of care to improve, health professionals and consumers need to know what should be done differently and how much of a difference is necessary to get a better result. This means that we need much more comprehensive measures of quality than are available routinely in any nation today. At the same time, we need to reexamine fundamentally the way medicine is practiced. Despite major differences in financing and spending levels across nations, regions, and health plans, there are vast similarities at the micro level in how health care is delivered. Electronic clinical information systems capable of tracking patients across multiple providers and settings of care are rare. Relatively little proactive management of preventive care and chronic disease occurs. Communication across the divide between primary and specialty care is limited. And the ability for people in any of these systems to match the array of what is possible against the needs of a particular patient is limited and rarely supported by modern decision support tools.

Medical science has progressed at a breathtaking rate. Yet fundamental changes in the way medical care is organized, managed, and delivered will be necessary if we are all to take advantage of what science has to offer. These changes must pursue four goals: better information, greater standardization, systems-level innovation, and real and rapid reform.

Today, there is a notable lack of an appropriate information infrastructure for delivering, evaluating, rewarding, or improving the delivery of health care services. It is not possible within today's information environment to routinely monitor performance on clinically detailed measures of technical quality or patient-centered care at all levels in the health care system. Much of the information content required to assess performance is also essential for managing the delivery of excellent, evidence-based care. Most programs in place today to profile physicians or medical groups, reward performance, create tiered networks, or provide public reports rely primarily on administrative data. These data sets are missing key information necessary for managing patients with complex chronic conditions. You cannot manage what you cannot measure. Until we solve the information infrastructure deficit, we can expect only limited progress on closing the quality gap.

We also need standardized approaches to delivering evidence-based or guideline-adherent care. Resistance to standardization in medical care delivery is substantial. The more standardized approaches are often dismissed by labeling them as "cookbook medicine." The detractors of standardization fail to acknowledge that if you have a good cookbook and follow the instructions, you can expect to achieve the intended outcome. We have a health care system today that is dominated by embracing exceptions rather than rules, and we have had little earnest discussion of the serious consequences of failing to standardize. In work done using the Assessing Care of Vulnerable Elders (ACOVE) system, a set of guidelines for care of older patients, a relationship was found between rates of adherence to the indicators and likelihood of survival in the subsequent three years. In that analysis, 28 percent of patients who received an average of 44 percent of recommended care died during the next three years compared with just 18 percent of patients who received an average of 62 percent of recommended care.[27] Standardization will require work, but it is essential.

Moreover, we also need systems-level innovation in health care delivery. It is common to think that the delivery of health care is a zero sum game — that improvement in one area must necessarily come at the expense of something else. If physicians are to deliver better care, in this view, they will have to work longer or harder (or we will have to train more physicians to do the work). Yet there is great potential for innovative strategies to result in improved care delivery within the current level of resource use — that is, working smarter, rather than longer.

A starting point is to identify the goals of health service delivery (for example, optimizing the quality of life for patients with chronic disease) and then the elements of care that are necessary to achieve those aims. Once the elements are identified, one can evaluate whether there are alternative ways to organize the delivery of health care (both the processes and who performs those processes) that could better achieve the goals. For example, some care can be delivered in groups rather than one-on-one (e.g., ongoing monitoring of care for chronic conditions such as diabetes or hypertension). Better information systems can reduce the need for certain tests (duplicate testing that gets done because the results have been lost or not transmitted from another provider) and the time required to collect data and incorporate that information into treatment planning. All of these approaches have been shown to be effective ways of delivering health services.

Above all, we need to act—and act now. The deficits in the performance of the health care system are enormous and the rate of change appears glacial. Finding ways to accelerate the rate of change is important. In doing this, we must identify tools that can be used by physicians in solo and small group practice as well as in integrated group practices. Most physicians practice in the former rather than the latter settings. If we are to improve the quality of care for the entire country, then strategies must meet the needs of those in different practice settings.

As the debate over health care reform goes forward, we should pay more attention to evidence and less to unsubstantiated worries. We should worry more about the unintended consequences—unnecessary death and disability—associated with our current approach to care delivery than the consequences of efforts to make things better. And while we are broadening coverage and seeking to contain costs, we should commit ourselves to investing in the research, technology, and institutional changes that can ensure our providers are delivering the high-quality health care that Americans deserve.

NOTES

1   T. F. Lyons and B. C. Payne, "The Quality of Physicians' Health-Care Performance: A Comparison Against Optimal Criteria for Treatment of the Elderly and Younger Adults in Community Hospitals," *JAMA* 227, no. 8 (February 25, 1974): 925–28.

2   E. A. McGlynn, S. M. Asch, J. Adams, J. Keesey, J. Hicks, A. DeCristofaro, and E. A. Kerr, "The Quality of Health Care Delivered to Adults in the United States," *New*

England Journal of Medicine 348, no. 26 (June 26, 2003): 2635–45; R. Mangione-Smith, A. H. DeCristofaro, C. M. Setodji, J. Keesey, D. J. Klein, J. A. Adams, M. A. Schuster, and E. A. McGlynn, "The Quality of Ambulatory Care Delivered to Children in the United States," *New England Journal of Medicine* 357, no. 15 (October 11, 2007): 1515–23.

3   E. A. McGlynn, "There Is No Perfect Health System," *Health Affairs* 23, no. 3 (May-June 2004): 100–2.

4   K. N. Lohr, R. H. Brook, C. J. Kamberg, G. A. Goldberg, A. Leibowitz, J. Keesey, D. Reboussin, and J. P. Newhouse, "Use of Medical Care in the Rand Health Insurance Experiment: Diagnosis- and Service-Specific Analyses in a Randomized Controlled Trial," *Medical Care* 24, no. 9 (September 1986): s1–87.

5   Robert J. Blendon, "Health Care in the 2008 Presidential Primaries," *New England Journal of Medicine* 358, no. 4 (January 24, 2008): 414–22.

6   Ibid.

7   K. Lohr, ed., *Medicare, A Strategy for Quality Assurance: A Report of a Study by a Committee of the Institute of Medicine* (Washington, DC: National Academy Press, 1990), 1:4.

8   Institute of Medicine, *Crossing the Quality Chasm: A New Health System for the 21st Century* (Washington, DC: National Academy Press, 2001), 232.

9   A. Donabedian, *The Definition of Quality and Approaches to Its Assessment* (Ann Arbor, MI: Health Administration Press, 1980).

10 M. A. Schuster, E. A. McGlynn, and R. H. Brook, "How Good Is the Quality of Health Care in the United States?" *Milbank Quarterly* 76, no. 4 (1998): 517–63.

11 E. A. McGlynn, E. A. Kerr, C. Damberg, and S. Asch, eds., *Quality of Care for Women: A Review of Selected Clinical Conditions and Quality Indicators* (Santa Monica, CA: RAND Corporation, MR-1284-HCFA, 2000); E. A. McGlynn, C. Damberg, E. Kerr, and M. Schuster, eds., *Quality of Care for Children and Adolescents: A Review of Selected Clinical Conditions and Quality Indicators* (Santa Monica, CA: RAND Corporation, MR-1283-HCFA, 2000); E. A. Kerr, S. Asch, E. G. Hamilton, and E. A. McGlynn, eds., *Quality of Care for Cardiopulmonary Conditions: A Review of the Literature and Quality Indicators* (Santa Monica, CA: RAND Corporation, MR-1282-AHRQ, 2000); E. A. Kerr, S. Asch, E. G. Hamilton, and E. A. McGlynn, eds., *Quality of Care for General Medical Conditions: A Review of the Literature and Quality Indicators* (Santa Monica, CA: RAND Corporation, MR-1280-AHRQ, 2000); S. Asch, E. A. Kerr, E. G. Hamilton, J. L. Reifel, and E. A. McGlynn, eds., *Quality of Care for Oncologic Conditions and HIV: A Review of the Literature and Quality Indicators* (Santa Monica, CA: RAND Corporation, MR-1281-AHRQ, 2000).

12 E. A. Kerr, E. A. McGlynn, J. Adams, J. Keesey, and S. M. Asch, "Profiling the Quality of Care in 12 Communities: Results from the CQI Study," *Health Affairs* 23, no. 3 (2004): 247–56.

13 J. W. Baker, M. Mellon, J. Wald et al., "A Multiple-Dosing, Placebo-Controlled Study of Budesonide Inhalation Suspension Given Once or Twice Daily for Treatment of Persistent Asthma in Young Children and Infants," *Pediatrics* 103 (1999): 414–21.

14 R. J. Adams, A. Fuhlbrigge, J. A. Finkelstein et al., "Impact of Inhaled Anti-Inflammatory Therapy on Hospitalization and Emergency Visits for Children with Asthma," *Pediatrics* 107 (2001): 706–11.

15 S. Suissa, P. Ernst, S. Benayoun, M. Baltzaan, and B. Cai, "Low-Dose Inhaled Corticosteroids and the Prevention of Death from Asthma," *New England Journal of Medicine* 343 (2000): 332–36.

16 P. Caione, M. Villa, N. Capozza, M. De Gennaro, and G. Rizzoni, "Predictive Risk Factors for Chronic Renal Failure in Primary High-Grade Vesico-Ureteric Reflux," *BJU International* 93 (2004): 1309–12.

17 Centers for Disease Control and Prevention, *Sexually Transmitted Disease Surveillance 2000* (Atlanta: Centers for Disease Control and Prevention, 2001).

18 D. Scholes, A. Stergachis, F. E. Heidrich et al., "Prevention of Pelvic Inflammatory Disease by Screening for Cervical Chlamydia Infection," *New England Journal of Medicine* 334 (1996): 1362–66.

19 P. S. Hussey et al. "How Does the Quality of Care Compare in Five Countries?" *Health Affairs* 23, no. 3 (2004): 96–97.

20 Ibid., 97.

21 R. H. Miller and H. S. Luft, "HMO Plan Performance Update: An Analysis of the Literature, 1997–2001," *Health Affairs* 21, no. 4 (July–August 2002): 63–86.

22 S. B. Soumerai, J. Avorn, D. Ross-Degnan, and S. Gortmaker, "Payment Restrictions for Prescription Drugs under Medicaid: Effects on Therapy, Cost, and Equity," *New England Journal of Medicine* 317, no. 9 (August 27, 1987): 550–56.

23 S. B. Soumerai, D. Ross-Degnan, S. Gortmaker, and J. Avorn, "Withdrawing Payment for Nonscientific Drug Therapy; Intended and Unexpected Effects of a Large-Scale Natural Experiment," *JAMA* 263, no. 6 (February 9, 1990): 831–39.

24 M. Schoenbaum, J. Unützer, D. McCaffrey, N. Duan, C. Sherbourne, and K. B. Wells, "The Effects of Primary Care Depression Treatment on Patients' Clinical Status and Employment," *Health Services Research* 37, no. 5 (October 2002): 1145–58.

25 Phillip Longman, "The Best Care Anywhere," *The Washington Monthly*, January/February 2005.

26 S.M. Asch, E.A. McGlynn, M.M. Hogan, R.A. Hayward, P. Shekelle, L. Ruben-
    stein, J. Keesey, J. Adams, and E.A. Kerr, "Comparison of Quality of Care for
    Patients in the Veterans Health Administration and Patients in a National Sam-
    ple," *Annals of Internal Medicine* 141, no. 12 (December 21, 2004): 938–45.

27 T. Higashi, P.G. Shekelle, J.L. Adams, C.J. Kamberg, C.P. Roth, D.H. Solomon,
    D.B. Reuben, L. Chiang, C.H. MacLean, J.T. Chang, R.T. Young, D.M. Saliba, and
    N.W. Wenger, "Quality of Care Is Associated with Survival in Vulnerable Older
    Patients," *Annals of Internal Medicine* 143, no. 4 (August 16, 2005): 274–81.

CHAPTER FIVE

The New Push for American Health Security

JACOB S. HACKER

In the spring of 1962, as Ray Charles's "Unchain My Heart" was climbing the singles charts, another recording by a noted performer was playing in American living rooms across the country. The words may not have been as catchy as Charles's, but they were no less urgent. The speaker on the vinyl LP warned about a bill before Congress that would bring about "socialized medicine" in the United States, imploring listeners to enlist their friends and neighbors to write in opposition:

> Write those letters now; call your friends, and tell them to write them. If you don't, this program, I promise you, will pass just as surely as the sun will come up tomorrow. And behind it will come federal programs that will invade every area of freedom as we have known it in this country. Until one day...we will awake to find that we have socialism. And if you don't do this, and I don't do it, one of these days you and I are going to spend our sunset years telling our children and our children's children what is was like in America when men were free.[1]

The voice, soon to be familiar in American political debates, was Ronald Reagan's. And the program sinisterly poised to steal our freedoms was Medicare—the popular federal health plan for the aged that passed in 1965.

As this little trip down memory lane suggests, Americans have been fighting over health care for a very long time. With pendulum-like regularity, the battle has flared up roughly fifteen years after it last flamed out. Reform efforts came to a halt in 1920, 1935, 1950, 1965 (when, despite Reagan's efforts, Medicare and Medicaid were enacted), 1980, and, of course, upon the crashing failure of the Clinton health plan in 1994.

Each time, well-intentioned reformers armed with the sorts of statistics and concerns so carefully laid out in the previous chapters of this volume have argued that change must finally come. And each time reformers have run headlong into a wall of ideologically charged opposition that has thrown exorbitant resources and energy into convincing political leaders and Americans that they will be made worse off by change.

To be sure, the predictions have not always been as dire as the loss of freedom foreseen by Reagan. Yet the charges have always involved the frightening claim that government involvement will lower the quality and raise the costs of medical care, threatening the wellness and financial security of those who are already insured. In a political culture skeptical of egalitarian government efforts and a political framework designed to make major policy transformation difficult, reform efforts have again and again collapsed under the weight of public concerns and interest-group opposition, leaving reformers short of their ultimate goal of universal health security.

So here we are in 2008, back on schedule to have a major national debate about health care, and with every right to ask: Why should anything be different this time? Is the present moment sufficiently more auspicious than when our leaders last waged battle on this issue? Has the line-up of contenders or the experiences or views of the public changed in fundamental ways? And what are the lessons those leaders should take from the past about the most feasible route to change today—particularly from the high-profile failure of the Clinton health plan in the early 1990s?

As the now-clichéd aphorism of George Santayana has it, those who do not learn from the mistakes of history are doomed to repeat them (or, he might have added, to come up with new mistakes of their own). But the lessons of the past are rarely as simple as we like to assume. Much of the social scientific analysis of health policy has been dominated by economists, whose methodological tools equip them well to examine the economic effects and incentives of existing and potential policies.

Economists have no special disciplinary claim, however, when it comes to political analysis and forecasting—the traditional domain of political scientists. Yet, for a variety of reasons, discussions of the elusive concept of "political feasibility" are today mostly dominated by those trained in economics. (One of these reasons is that surprisingly few political scientists actually study the political formation and effects of public policy.)[2] In what follows, therefore, I bring the insights of political science to bear on the question of whether and under what circumstances major reform of American health care might occur in the relatively near future.

This analysis demonstrates that some of the greatest political barriers to change of the past have weakened: a business community willing to throw in its lot with private bargaining and benefits, whatever the cost; a labor movement torn by its continuing faith in union-negotiated welfare capitalism; and, above all, a robust public confidence that private health insurance will inevitably expand. Alongside these long-term developments, moreover, new strategic thinking is taking place among reformers about how, in light of recent defeats, their long-deferred goal might yet be achieved. Central to this thinking is a recognition that the biggest political challenge is how to deal with America's eroding yet entrenched employment-based framework of insurance in a way that is sensitive to the easily ignited fears of well-insured workers that they will be asked to pay more for less.

And yet, the long arc of American political history also reveals newly potent barriers, barriers that guarantee the fight will be bitter, the stakes epic, and the outcome deeply uncertain. The most dramatic of these obstacles, the hyperpolarization of American politics and the erosion of public faith in politics and government, suggest that constructively channeling the debate over health reform into concrete achievements will be one of the greatest tests our democratic process has faced—and one it may not pass.

EXPLAINING THE DISTINCTIVENESS OF U.S. HEALTH POLICY

To start our exploration, it is worth asking a deceptively simple question: Why is the United States the only rich democracy without guaranteed health coverage for all (or virtually all)? Although the health policies found in other affluent nations are often bafflingly complex and diverse, this complexity and diversity mask substantial similarity across rich democracies' health programs, virtually all of which share two bedrock characteristics: they cover all citizens, and they employ measures to contain costs at a high level of aggregation.[3] Against this "international standard" (as Joseph White nicely calls it), only the United States looks like a conspicuous outlier, its public programs covering less than half the population, its overall spending largely unconstrained.[4]

As Table 5.1 shows, America's distinctive position cannot easily be chalked up to the penuriousness of its government. Yes, public health insurance in the United States covers just over 27 percent of Americans, whereas virtually all other rich nations cover their entire citizenry (column 1). But because American medical costs are so much higher than health costs in other nations (column 2), total U.S. public spending on health care per capita (including tax breaks for coverage and coverage for public employees) is actually the highest in the world (column 3). As the fourth column of the table shows, moreover, U.S. health spending (both public and private) is also growing much more quickly. What is distinctive, however, is that a very large share of the United States' very high spending is financed by voluntary private health insurance, sponsored by employers and heavily (and regressively) subsidized by the federal government through the tax code. (In 2004, the cost of exempting health benefits from taxation in terms of forgone tax revenues was $188.5 billion, with nearly 27 percent of this benefit going to the 16 percent of the population with annual family incomes in excess of $100,000.) This point holds more generally: Private employment-based benefits (mainly health insurance and retirement pensions) play a much larger role in the United States than other rich nations — so much more so that, as the final column of Table 5.1 shows, accounting for these private benefits raises U.S. spending on health and economic security as a share of the economy to something close to the average for advanced industrial democracies.

Nor, as Jill Quadagno and Brandon McKelvey show in their chapter of this book, is it simply the case that proposals for universal health care never made it to the top of the agenda of American politics. On the contrary: Presidents Truman, Nixon, Carter, and, of course, Clinton all made high-profile pushes for national reform. In each case, however, universal insurance for working-age Americans failed to win out. Why?

COUNTRY	SHARE OF POPULATION COVERED BY GOVERNMENT HEALTH PROGRAMS (2004)	TOTAL GOVERNMENT & PRIVATE HEALTH SPENDING PER CAPITA (2004)	GOVERNMENT HEALTH SPENDING PER CAPITA, INCLUDING TAX BREAKS (1998/99)	ANNUAL MEDICAL INFLATION IN EXCESS OF POPULATION GROWTH & AGING (1985–2002)	PUBLIC & PRIVATE SPENDING ON HEALTH & ECONOMIC SECURITY AFTER TAXES AS A SHARE OF GDP (2001)
Australia	100%	$3120	$1300	.88%	24.0%
Austria	98%	$3124		.65%	24.8%
Belgium	99%	$3044		1.1%	26.3%
Canada	100%	$3165	$1500	.43%	23.3%
Denmark	100%	$2881		-.10%	26.4%
Finland	100%	$2235		-.43%	22.6%
France	99.9%	$3159	$1400	.61%	31.2%
Germany	89.8%	$3043	$1600	.76%	30.8%
Greece	100%	$2162		1.31%	
Iceland	100%	$331		1.52%	21.7%
Ireland	100%	$2596		-.65%	13.9%
Italy	100%	$2467	$1150		25.3%
Japan	100%	$2249	$1200	-.03%	22.1%
Netherlands	62.5%	$3041		.88%	25.0%
New Zealand	100%	$2083			18.2%
Norway	100%	$3966		1.50%	23.6%
Spain		$2094		1.25%	18.9%
Sweden	100%	$2825	$1300	.19%	30.6%
Switzerland	100%	$4077	$2100	1.88%	
United Kingdom	100%	$2508	$1100	1.43%	27.1%
Non-US average	97.3%	$2859	$1405.5	.73%	24.2%
United States	27.3%	$6102	$2500	2%	24.5%

Sources: *OECD Health Data 2007*, "Share of population eligible for a defined set of health care goods and services under public programmes," (Paris: OECD, 2008); Gerard F. Anderson, Bianca K. Frogner, and Uwe E. Reinhardt, "Health Spending in OECD Countries in 2004: An Update," *Health Affairs*, September/October 2007; 26(5): 1481–1489; Steffie Woolhandler and David U. Himmelstein, "Paying for National Health Insurance—and Not Getting It," *Health Affairs*, July/August 2002; 21(4): 88–98; Chapin White, "Health Care Spending Growth: How Different Is the United States from the Rest of the OECD?" *Health Affairs*, January/February 2007; 26(1):154–161; Willem Adema and Maxime Ladaique, "Net Social Expenditure, 2005," OECD Social, Employment, and Migration Working Papers, No. 29 (Paris: OECD, 2005), available online at http://www.oecd.org/dataoecd/56/2/35632106.pdf.

Table 5.1   American health care and social policy in cross-national relief

The beginning of an answer is the observation that political parties have historically differed on the proper role of government in medical care. In cross-national research, a well-supported finding is that rule by parties of the left, particularly during the formative years of welfare state development, is associated with more expansive and generous social programs.[5]

The United States, of course, has one of the weakest traditions of socialism and social democracy of any rich democracy. Unions in the United States have relatively limited scope (and much reduced scope today, when they represent less than 12.5 percent of all workers, and just over 8 percent of private-sector workers). Moreover, true parties of the left have never been able to gain a foothold in America's strong two-party structure, both because of the weakness of organized labor and the difficulties that third parties face in America's winner-take-all electoral system.

Leftist rule is certainly not a necessary condition for universal health care, as it has been adopted under governments of varying partisan stripes. But it does appear strongly associated with the establishment of comprehensive "national health services" — programs in which hospitals are owned by government and doctors receive a government salary. More generally, extended governance by socialist and social democratic parties is associated with a diminished role for private insurance and direct consumer payments, which the left has long viewed as inegalitarian.[6] Again, the United States stands out even among other English-speaking nations as distinctively hostile territory for left parties, and as the affluent nation most reliant on private insurance and out-of-pocket spending.

In all nations, however, the scope for political leaders to achieve their favored goals is heavily constrained by the structure of political institutions, particularly the opportunities for blocking activity that institutions create for powerful opponents of national health programs like the medical profession. As Ellen Immergut has convincingly argued, opponents of large-scale government entry into the health field have generally been advantaged when a polity has a large number of "veto points," such as federalism and a separation of powers between the executive and legislature.[7] This no doubt helps explain why no nation with federalism (partially autonomous subnational governments, like the American states or Canadian provinces) has adopted a national health service; why across nations the share of medical spending financed by government is strongly correlated with the number of institutional veto points; and why Switzerland, with its strong federalism and tradition of the use of popular referenda by organized groups, has long been characterized by the most anemic government role in health policy of all European nations. It is also consistent with the fact that the United States — which, with its separation of legislative and executive powers and federalist structure, has the most veto-point-ridden polity of any rich democracy—remains the only advanced industrial state that does not have a broad framework of public coverage or cost containment and relies principally on voluntary employment-based coverage.[8]

Still, with the exception of the United States, all advanced industrial democracies have adopted some version of the international standard. This suggests that institutional barriers are better at slowing than halting government's entry into the medical field. The timing and sequence of policy interventions, however, may be highly consequential for the *form* that national health policies ultimately take. Most countries began to intrude into the doctor-patient relationship by subsidizing nongovernmental insurers, rather than financing services. These policies created important vested interests in a pluralist financing structure and reinforced doctors' preferences for fee-for-service payment. How extensive and long-lived these arrangements were thus had crucial effects on the types of systems countries ended up with.[9] Countries in which authoritative government action to consolidate or supplant nongovernmental insurance took longer to achieve generally ended up with more decentralized and costly health financing systems in which private insurance and finance played a more pivotal role—in part because delay allowed the formation and enrichment of a formidable collection of private stakeholders, and in part because sophisticated private care represents such a massive burden for government budgets to assume.

This is a paradigm example of what social scientists call *path dependence*, temporal processes in which early choices create self-reinforcing effects that are inherently difficult to reverse.[10] The United States, again, represents an extreme case: Private insurance has, in effect, come to play the role that public programs do elsewhere, and this role has proved as difficult to dislodge as the public foundations of mature welfare states.[11] At the most basic level, the answer to the question of why the United States lacks national health insurance is that *Americans have come to rely on predominantly private sources of health security*. To be sure, private coverage is contracting, and many who have private coverage are insufficiently protected against ruinous financial losses. It remains the case, however, that private insurance reaches just over three in five nonelderly Americans. And this means, in turn, that proposals for public coverage face singular hurdles—not just the opposition of a huge and resourceful private medical sector, but also the fears of privately insured Americans about threats to existing protections.

ROOTS OF AMERICAN EXCEPTIONALISM

Now deeply embedded, America's unique reliance on the private sector for health security was hardly foreordained. It emerged from political conflicts in which outcomes could have been different. Nor was it guaranteed by the early defeat of public coverage. Endemically prone to failure, the private insurance market had to be actively constructed by private leadership and public policy, which came together at critical junctures in the early to mid-twentieth century to bolster private institutions as a bulwark against state intervention.

The crucial interlude was the 1940s through the late 1950s—often seen as merely the calm eddy between the two "big bangs" of American welfare-state building: the New Deal and the Great Society. The standard narrative about this period highlights the blocking role played by Southern Democrats, who dominated leadership positions in Congress thanks to the lack of effective partisan competition in the South. To limit the reach of the federal government into local arrangements of racial hierarchy and exclusion, many Southern Democrats aligned with Republicans against new social policy initiatives, including national health insurance. Yet important policy departures took place despite the stalemate over national reform, and the success of opponents of national health insurance rested critically on promoting a credible private alternative, frequently with extensive government assistance.

During the debate over national health insurance in the late 1940s, for example, the American Medical Association (AMA) made voluntary health insurance the foundation of its bitter assault. Emphasizing that "[y]ou can't beat something with nothing," the AMA's PR guru declared: "We want everybody in the health insurance field selling insurance as he never sold it before. If we can get ten million more people insured in the next year and ten million more in the next year, the threat of socialized medicine in this country will be over."[12]

Although the AMA was the most prominent group touting the virtues of private insurance, it was hardly alone. Commercial insurers were also on board, of course, and so too was corporate America. Large employers backed private benefits as a means of buying workers' good-will, placating (or heading off) unions, and undercutting Democratic efforts to enact national health insurance. In 1949, *Life* magazine wryly described workplace fringe benefits as "ransom devices to buy off the Welfare State" — a ransom that would become more and more dear as coverage spread and health care costs rose.

Indeed, once the floodgates of private provision opened, even orga-nized labor joined the bandwagon. When, for example, the Eisenhower administration announced it was reviewing the tax treatment of health insurance in 1954, the Congress of Industrial Organizations (CIO) sub-mitted a confidential memo on behalf of "five million wage earners" in support of the tax exemption of insurance.[13] Though the CIO noted the huge new levies on workers with private insurance that would result if health benefits were taxed, its main warning concerned "the harmful effect which a reversal of the present tax ruling would have on the growth of voluntary hospitalization and medical plans."[14] The same CIO that had stated in 1949 that "[t]he voluntary groups are limited by their very nature from providing comprehensive care to everyone" now criticized any action that would "adversely affect the continued growth of volun-tary prepayment plans...as a mechanism for providing comprehensive health services to the American people."[15]

The spread of private benefits into the workforce had two far-reaching political effects. The first was to displace the battle for national health insurance into the areas where private benefits remained rare: namely, among the aged and the very poor. In this light, Medicare and Medicaid — far from the precedents for universal coverage — were gap-filling measures that lessened pressure for national insurance by dealing with the groups most conspicuously left out of the private system.

This brings us to the second effect of the ascendance of private coverage: to create powerful, enduring hurdles to an expanded public role. Americans came to depend on the private system, and powerful vested interest arose within and around it. Major legislative changes to that system, even changes that would make Americans as a whole better off, increasingly ran headlong into the specific dislocations that reforms threatened. Just as with well-entrenched public programs like Medicare and Social Security, radically transforming established networks of private social provision is a political fool's errand. In this broader historical view, the failure of the Clinton health plan in the early 1990s was as much a reflection of the inherited barriers created by past policy battles as it was of the distinctive character of U.S. politics in *fin de siècle* America.

THE RISE AND DEMISE OF THE CLINTON HEALTH PLAN

Without too much simplification, American health care debates can be divided into two broad eras: the era of expansion, in which private and public coverage extended to reach ever more Americans, and the era of contraction, dating roughly to the late 1970s, when, as Katherine Swartz documents in her chapter in this book, coverage began its contemporary slide.

The debate over the Clinton health plan was the first to take place in this second era, and to the many who engaged in it, the urgency of the discussion was a direct reflection of worsening conditions on the ground. Surely, now that coverage was eroding, the United States would finally wake from its slumber and end its singular status as the only rich democracy reliant on voluntary, employer-provided health insurance to cover (or not, as the case often was) all but the poorest of its working-age citizens.

It did not work out that way, of course. The Health Security Act—1,342 pages long and based on an intricately complicated theory known as "managed competition within a budget"—was dead on arrival. But it succumbed not to some inexorable law of politics that makes any government attempt to deal with the problems in health insurance an impossible sell. Rather, it was an already-crippled creature dropped into the den of wolves that America's ultraexpensive medical complex had spawned.

First were the self-inflicted wounds. Rather than press for quick action based on broad principles, Clinton's policy team constructed a grandiose process for developing an ideal plan that could bridge all the major ideological and political divides. Rather than build on existing programs, insiders in the process denigrated them as flawed and insufficient. One memo on Medicare by a top architect of the Clinton plan declared, for example, that "Medicare's entire history should be a lesson on how not to structure a national health program," ignoring that Medicare was the only national program the United States had and one that was overwhelmingly popular.[16]

At the root of the problem was the elevation of policy analysis over political analysis, a persistent problem for progressive reformers but one abetted in recent decades by the rise of a much more sophisticated science of policy development. As anyone who attempts to follow health policy discussions knows, health reform has become an arcane arena of dueling statistics and approaches. And as anyone who attempted to follow them in the early 1990s will recall, the Clinton plan was formulated in this hothouse of competing reform "models."[17] Even the unwieldy moniker of Clinton's hybrid approach, "managed competition within a budget," belied the plan's aspiration to bridge the elite divide by synthesizing articulated reform visions (private plan competition, public insurance with a cap on spending) embodying sharply contrasting assumptions but sharing the same commitment to technically minded policy analysis.

All this may seem to make too much of elite discourse. But consider the Clinton administration's missteps in light of the policy-analytic mindset. In the craft of policy design, the plan was a tour de force, envisioning the comprehensive remaking of America's medical-industrial complex. Existing employment-based health plans? Inadequate and destructive of the delicate incentives the plan envisioned. The answer: let only the largest corporations run their own plans under strict rules, a choice that leading employer representatives decried as "movement toward a government financed and controlled system."[18] No platform for properly incentivized consumer choice? Build it, in the form of so-called Health Alliances, a new nation-spanning administrative infrastructure, and the plans will come. And the plans? HMOs and other tightly managed products were the wave of the future, so make these the centerpiece, regardless of the fears they might provoke. The architect of Medicare, Wilbur Cohen, liked to say that social reform was 1 percent inspiration and 99 percent implementation. The Clinton plan was 99 percent inspiration.

The problem was not that the Clinton reformers did not have a strategy to enact their proposal. The problem was that the strategy was their proposal. As a task force memo by Walter Zelman, a central formulator of the plan, put it in March 1993, "We have found a unique blend of approaches that is better than competing models.... It is not a low-level compromise, a product of political give and take, but a genuinely higher synthesis.... We have something...we can really be proud of—a true political breakthrough, and [a] new possibility of achieving the kind of consensus we've never gotten to before."[19] The proposal was the political breakthrough.

It was but a short distance from there to the denigration of existing institutions as flawed and inefficient means of achieving "a genuinely higher synthesis," no matter their familiarity or entrenchment. And it was but a short distance from there to the conceit that coalition building was mostly a matter of policy fine-tuning, of brokering political deals ex ante via the fine points of policy blueprints. But it was a very long distance from there to a proposal that could address public concerns about declining coverage and rising costs without stoking fear or confusion. Premised on resolving elite-level disagreement, the structural details of the proposal were not just incomprehensible to most Americans but frankly threatening, envisioning the near-total eclipse of employment-based insurance and the massive expansion of tightly managed plans. The resulting scheme was so complicated, so intricate, so unwieldy it could be portrayed as anything opponents wanted, and fearsome caricatures of liberty-robbing, big-government monstrosities were soon unleashed — caricatures that could scarcely be dispelled with vague mantras of "choice," "security," "simplicity," and "savings." Not surprisingly, public support for the plan plummeted after Clinton's stirring September 1993 speech describing the proposal.

Hobbled, the plan was then crushed under the weight of interest-group and conservative resistance. It had tried to appease all the major groups. The problem was that all these groups still had plenty of incentive to fight, and plenty of money and other resources to wage that fight. No other nation has tried to transform a medical-industrial complex as large or as a costly as the American system, or to do so as thoroughly. Once the battle heated up, even ordinary Americans sympathetic to the cause grew wary, fearful they would lose their own benefits without something better in return. Born in a policy hothouse, the plan wilted in the cold winds of politics, friendless, misunderstood, and shunned by the very middle-class Americans whose plight had prompted the effort.

IS THE TIME NOW RIPE?

Should we expect a different response this time around? There is no question that health security has eroded since the Clinton health plan's defeat. Personal bankruptcies caused by medical costs, rampant unin-surance and underinsurance, runaway medical debt, crippling benefit costs — all these problems have grown more prevalent and troubling, and all of them increasingly affect the politically crucial middle class. As Katherine Swartz's chapter in this book vividly demonstrates, the ranks of the uninsured have grown substantially since the early 1990s — among the middle class as well as lower income groups (even though the poor-est of Americans have been cushioned by the major expansion of public coverage for low-income groups). Medical bankruptcy, as Elizabeth War-ren and Deborah Thorne show, is also a major, troubling, and almost certainly growing problem — one that affects those who have health cov-erage as well as those without it.

Indeed, if the overriding problem of the 1990s was lack of health insurance — a problem that has, of course, worsened — the looming prob-lem of this decade may well be "underinsurance," the lack of *adequate* health insurance. In the twelve months prior to May 2007, according to a survey by *Consumer Reports,* around three in ten nonelderly adults who had health insurance lacked adequate coverage.[20] Nearly six in ten of the underinsured postponed needed medical care because of the cost, nearly four in ten had to put off home or car maintenance or repairs due to medical expenses, a third had to dig deep into their savings to pay for medical care, and more than one in five made job-related decisions based mainly on their health care needs. Strikingly, the median family income of the underinsured was $58,000 — almost exactly the same as the median income of those with adequate coverage. The underinsured are just as likely to be white as the well-insured, nearly as well educated, and just as likely to work full-time and in large or medium-sized compa-nies. The only consistent way in which they differed from those who are better protected is that they were at grave, and growing, economic risk.

The main reason for these worrisome trends is simple: As medical costs and health premiums continue to skyrocket, traditional employ-ment-based coverage is declining. Some surveys suggest its reach has plummeted by as much as 9 percentage points between 2000 and 2005, while others indicate a steadier and somewhat smaller drop.[21] What is not in dispute is that Americans are ever less likely to be covered by their employers, and that employers are asking workers to pay a larger share of the cost of their coverage and care. With health premiums growing by roughly 50 percent in inflation-adjusted terms between 2000 and 2006, over a period in which the typical family's income actually declined, it is little surprise that health care costs and coverage have risen in prominence as stated concerns of Americans in opinion surveys.[22]

What the failure of the Clinton health plan vividly demonstrates, however, is that most Americans—even the underinsured and soon-to-be-uninsured, the potentially uninsurable and the one-illness-from-bankrupt—can be scared into fearing that changing America's inadequate public-private patchwork means higher costs and lower quality. This is the legacy of an insurance structure that lulls many into believing they are secure when they are not, that hides vast costs in quiet deductions from workers' pay, that leaves government paying the tab for the most vulnerable and the least well, and that so fragments the purchase of care that no one can bargain for lower prices or judge the value of what is being bought. Call it the catch-22 of health reform: It is the very failings of our insurance system that make dealing with those failings so devilishly hard.

Historically, advocates of reform have looked at this challenge through a rationalist lens, assuming that the basic problem is showing Americans that their fears of higher costs and lower quality due to reform are ungrounded. The evidence for such a demonstration is certainly easy to come by. With regard to costs, the United States not only spends much more than any other nation (either per capita or as a share of the economy), but has also seen its spending grow much more quickly than the norm for other rich democracies since the mid-1980s (refer back to Table 5.1). And one does not need to look abroad to see the cost-control advantages of public insurance: Since the introduction of cost controls in the 1980s, Medicare's expenditures have grown substantially slower than private insurance spending.[23]

If the assertion that greater government involvement inevitably drives up costs crumbles in the face of the cross-national and historical evidence, more plausible is the common claim that America's high level of spending guarantees much better care than seen abroad—care that would be made dramatically worse, or so the argument continues, by increased government involvement. But the growing body of research on health quality and outcomes has not been particularly kind to this claim either.

For starters, the dramatically lower spending seen abroad does not seem to be due mainly to "rationing." Waiting lists do crop up in other rich nations, but even countries without waiting lists spend much less than we do. The United States has fewer doctors, hospital beds, and nurses per person than the norm, and Americans (while less healthy overall) visit doctors and hospitals less often and have shorter hospital stays. Even the prevalence of high-tech equipment like MRIs does not look exceptionally high. And the United States lags far behind other rich nations in the use of information technology to improve quality.

Instead, the main reason for the United States' higher spending appears to be the high prices charged for our medical goods and services — the same medical goods and services that are delivered abroad. Add to this big price disparity the very high administrative costs of our fragmented system, and it becomes easier to understand how the United States can spend so much more with so little evidence of superior care.[24] In 2007, a team at the business consulting firm McKinsey & Company underook a comprehensive cross-national analysis of U.S. health spending. Their conclusion was that the United States spent almost a third more than would be expected based simply on the nation's per capita income — roughly $500 billion in extra spending a year — and that the modestly poorer health of Americans could not explain much of the difference. The principal reasons for the discrepancy, they concludeed, were higher input costs, especially higher drug costs; higher profits and taxes due to the heavy reliance on for-profit providers and insurers; and higher administrative costs. "Despite higher costs," the McKinsey team concluded, "the United States does not deliver objectively better quality and access for U.S. citizens as a whole relative to peer countries."[25]

Indeed, as David Meltzer, Elizabeth A. McGlynn and I show in the previous chapter, on some measures our care looks surprisingly substandard. For example, a recent six-country study concludes that "the U.S. scores particularly poorly on its ability to promote healthy lives, and on the provision of care that is safe and coordinated."[26] Meanwhile, analyses of "amenable mortality" — deaths that could have been prevented with timely care — find that the United States has the highest rate of preventable death before age seventy-five among rich nations, and that it is falling farther and farther behind.[27] To be sure, the United States performs well in some areas of high-tech care, as well as some areas of preventive screening; but given how much the United States spends, it is striking how poor American care often is.

Findings like these, published in highly respected journals of health care, provide firm grounding for believing that expanding health coverage through an increased government role is likely to reduce, rather than accelerate, the growth of costs, and improve, rather than harm, the overall quality of care—not least because of the extension of coverage to tens of millions of people whose insurance is inadequate, episodic, or nonexistent.

Yet advocates of fundamental change should be wary of the conceit that simply "getting the facts out" will spur a groundswell of public support for action or easily defuse the inevitable attacks on reform. Recent political science and behavioral psychology research suggests that when political appeals are highly emotional and personal—as, necessarily, are discussions of health care—voters are swayed by their immediate "gut" responses as much as, if not more than, by cognitive evaluation of the competing merits of alternative positions.[28] This is certainly one reason why initially strong public support for the Clinton health plan eroded, as critics pilloried the plan, often deploying grossly exaggerated or inaccurate claims designed to produce visceral reactions. And it suggests that reformers should be proactive in identifying and protecting the soft underbellies of their cause, as well as in thinking carefully about the nature of the public concerns to which they are responding.

WHAT AMERICANS THINK ABOUT REFORM

Public opinion regarding health care is notoriously tricky to interpret. Most Americans, for example, express satisfaction with their personal health care even as they voice high levels of dissatisfaction with the American "health system" as a whole. (Similarly split responses can be seen in evaluations of public school teachers and public schools as a whole, and members of Congress and Congress as a whole.) Moreover, responses to health care questions, like responses to other survey questions, are highly influenced by question wording, and there are many badly worded questions asked about health policy. Thus, the result of any one survey should be viewed with considerable skepticism; the strongest judgments come from analysis of survey questions that have been asked repeatedly in the same basic way over a fairly lengthy period of time.

The response to these sorts of survey questions suggests four broad conclusions about the public's views of health care reform and their evolution over time:

1. Health care is a leading concern of Americans, consistently at or near the top of private financial worries and less consistently but still quite frequently one of the major problems that Americans say face the nation. Public concern about health care as a national political issue appears to track elite debate closely, but whether it drives or follows national discussions is not entirely clear. Health care tends to emerge as a leading issue among the public during periods of heightened economic distress. As it rises as a concern, political efforts to address it amplify public identification of the issue as a major national priority, transforming private worries into a top-tier public issue.

2. Americans are generally supportive of covering the uninsured — even if doing so requires additional resources. Although survey questions on this topic that have been asked identically over time are less common than one might think, those repeated questions that do exist suggest that the level of support for government action to universalize coverage is roughly as high as it was in the early 1990s, with two-thirds of the public expressing approval. Support remains strong even when respondents are asked whether they would be willing to pay more to cover everyone, and far exceeds support for extending the tax cuts of 2001 and 2003, among respondents of all partisan leanings.[29] Figures 5.1 and 5.2 summarize the responses to two relevant questions from the General Social Survey: "Should government spend more or less on health care, given spending more implies an increase in your taxes?"; and "Is it the responsibility of government or people themselves to pay for doctor and hospital bills?" As can be seen, support for increased spending has risen fairly consistently since the mid-1980s. Support for government help with health care (as opposed to self-reliance) has fluctuated up and down but is higher now than at any point since the early 1970s, with the exception of the spike in support for government assistance in the years leading up to the debate over the Clinton health plan.

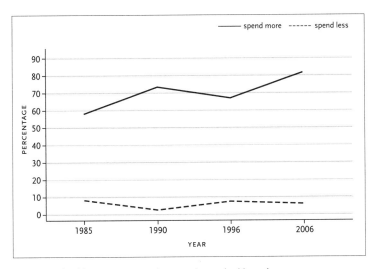

Figure 5.1 Should government spend more or less on health care?

[Source: General Social Survey, Question 1180, "Should government spend more or less on healthcare, given spending more implies an increase in your taxes?"]

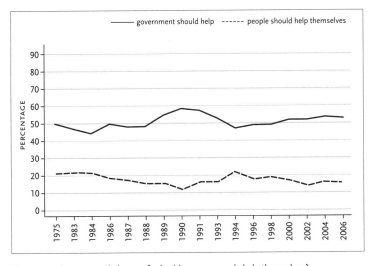

Figure 5.2 Government helps pay for health care or people help themselves?

[Source: General Social Survey, Question 311, "In general, some people think that it is the responsibility of the government in Washington to see to it that people have help in paying for doctors and hospital bills. Others think that these matters are not the responsibility of the federal government and that people should take care of these things themselves. Where would you place yourself on this scale, or haven't you made up your mind on this?" Responses 1 and 2 on the five-point scale are coded as "government should help"; responses 4 and 5 as "people should help themselves." "Agree with both" and no answer excluded.]

3. Public support for government action is coupled with substantial skepticism about the capacity of government, particularly when it comes to safeguarding the quality of medical care. Public trust in government has plummeted in the last generation, reaching a post-World War II nadir in the 1990s, climbing in the wake of the terrorist attacks of September 11, 2001, then falling again to 1990s levels by 2007.[30] Although supportive of government efforts to achieve universal coverage, most Americans express little confidence that government action will reduce their own costs, and a plurality generally state that private insurance would provide better quality care than government insurance. This makes it all the more remarkable how supportive of reform Americans are, but also suggests that public support is highly vulnerable to critics' charge that government involvement will drive up costs and degrade the quality of care.

4. Americans do not have firm opinions regarding the competing reform options about which policy experts so strenuously argue. Given multiple choices, they almost always split relatively evenly among them, and support for different options varies greatly with question wording. Nonetheless, the strongest support can consistently be elicited for measures requiring employers to provide health insurance to their workers. American are more ambivalent about both a national health program in which the federal government pays for care and measures to require individuals to purchase health insurance on their own. Despite decades of rhetoric criticizing government price restrictions and suggesting that patients should be more exposed to health costs, Americans are supportive of government cost controls for prescription drugs and medical services, believe that doctors and hospitals should be limited from charging "too much," and are wary of proposals that would increase out-of-pocket health spending.[31]

In all four of these areas, the relative stability of public opinion is more striking than its evolution. Recent public opinion on health care looks remarkably similar to the contours of opinion in the early 1990s, when health care reform emerged as a leading issue. Today, as then, support for major policy change is substantial—much higher than it is on many other issue where politicians have obliged by enacting legislative responses. Moreover, there is good reason to think that the dynamics of opinion are even more favorable for change today. The Clinton reform effort was launched amid a relatively conservative era in public opinion— a reality that became clearer when Republicans captured Congress in the wake of the Clinton health plan's failure. Over the last five to seven years, however, indices of public opinion show a significant move in a more liberal and pro-Democratic direction.[32] Americans are more likely to endorse a social safety net and express concern about rising economic inequality than they were when President George W. Bush took office, and much more likely to identify with the Democratic Party.

STRATEGIC SHIFTS IN FAVOR OF REFORM

But American politics is never simply about solving recognized problems, even when they affect a growing share of the middle class. The collapse of America's rickety public-private system has been predicted many times, and each time it has continued to limp along, hemorrhaging dollars, enrollees, and good will, yet still maintaining crucial reservoirs of support. Ultimately, then, three developments at the level of political elites may prove even more pivotal in improving the prospects for change.

The first is that corporate America may well be ready, after years of a promised conversion, to acquiesce to major changes. Although many corporate leaders favored action in the early 1990s—at least until the Clinton plan came out, medical inflation abetted, and Republican leaders and health industry interests cross-pressured them—even more today seem to recognize that absent action, they will increasingly be caught between the rock of rising costs and the hard place of hurting their workers by dropping coverage or providing bare-bones plans. The last decade has seen large employers pull out every trick in their arsenal for controlling costs, to little avail. Now, the only surefire way to cut expenses is to trim coverage and shift risks onto workers, which is not just unpalatable, but also likely to stoke public interest in reform.

The cause of reform would be greatly advantaged by weakened business resistance, but this outcome is by no means foreordained. In the early 1990s, a number of large unionized employers vocally supported national action, but their voices were drowned out by the fierce attacks of small employers and the growing wariness of less cost-pressed employers and their national representative organizations. Moreover, as Quadagno and McKelvey point out in their chapter, the next big thing for employers seeking to control health costs may well be "consumer directed health care," and in particular the move toward "defined-contribution" health plans that cap employers' obligations. Although the predicted mass movement in this direction has yet to materialize, surveys of corporations indicate that they believe that greatly increased cost sharing can control costs. As in the early 1990s, when employers opted for managed care as a putative private solution to runaway costs, reformers today may well be in a race against time, seeking to promote a reform vision that will split or placate the business community before a widespread employer turn toward private-sector solutions.

The second important development is a subtle but promising shift in the stance of organized labor. In the early 1990s, leading unions were deeply split over the appropriate course on health care, and a substantial number still clung to the notion that generous union-negotiated benefits could be sustained against the tide of economic transformation and business resistance. Today, there is both greater boldness and greater pragmatism, born of realism about the health of employment-based benefits and of desperation about a shrinking membership. Labor leaders know their movement's future rests on getting health care right, and that means moving beyond the current system.

The most visible figure in this shift is Andrew Stern, head of the Service Employees International Union (SEIU), as well as a leader of Change to Win—a coalition of unions that broke from the AFL-CIO in 2005. Stern is scathing in his denunciation of employment-based health insurance, which is particularly hard to secure for the nearly two million service workers SEIU represents (and even harder to secure for the unorganized service workers SEUI hopes to recruit). Yet Stern has proved willing to join with business leaders to call for intermediate steps toward universal insurance. The most notable alliance brought together Stern and the CEO of the union-disparaged retailer Wal-Mart, H. Lee Scott, who together vowed action on health care in the next five years. If history is any guide, these alliances are unlikely to last once the debate over reform heats up. But they are indicative of Stern's willingness to join forces with business leaders when he believes it can advance the cause of action. "We're way past the question, 'Can an employer solve this problem?'" Stern said in 2007. "We're at a point where the country has to solve the problem."[33]

The split within labor's ranks, however, suggests the limits of unions' influence. Once covering more than a third of the workforce, American unions now cover less than one tenth of private-sector workers (and around one in eight workers overall). In terms of their ability to spend on political campaigns and lobbying efforts, unions pale in influence compared to the other major players in health care: insurers, pharmaceutical companies, and business. But organized labor has arguably become more politically and organizationally adept since the health reform debate of the early 1990s. As Stern's leadership suggests, unions are less likely than they were in the past to worry about the effect of reform on negotiated private plans. And they clearly recognize that the next health reform debate may be their last real chance to free unions (and employers) from the heavy burden and constant struggle created by private health benefits for an aging unionized workforce.

This brings us to the final promising sign: the evolving strategies of advocates of comprehensive reform, who have returned to their field of dreams with greater sensitivity to some of the political risks they face—particularly the concern of Americans that their current coverage, however substandard, will be hurt or taken away without something better taking its place.

NEW DEBATE, NEW STRATEGIES

As the dismal failure of the Clinton health plan suggests, the two greatest barriers to reform are fear and financing—the fear that good employment-based coverage will be destroyed, and the substantial government financing (and taxes) that will be required to substitute public spending for the private spending that now runs through employers, largely in the hidden form of forgone cash wages of employees. Although Americans are much more supportive of government action to fix health care than conventional wisdom suggests, the Achilles' heel of reform is that most Americans do have some source of insurance most of the time. Against this backdrop, the easiest way to kill reform is to say, "Oh yes, I support change, but this change will destroy what you have, this change will make you pay more for less."

As we have seen, Americans are much more receptive than the conventional wisdom suggests to an enlarged government role in health care, including new taxes to support it.[34] But this is before the fear-mongering has really begun. Expanding public coverage may be the most promising route to cost control, but public coverage requires money, and money requires taxes, and taxes are politically difficult to enact even under the best of circumstances—not least when they substitute for the much less visible drain on workers' paychecks created by employment-based insurance.

When the rhetoric heats up, reformers will need to be able to fight fear with fear—the fear of government with the fear of losing private coverage, the fear of taxes with the fear of medical bankruptcy and debt. Reformers will also need to be able to fight fear with hope: with a clear, simple, and unthreatening vision that builds on what exists and meets public concerns head on—a vision that may lack the intellectual satisfaction of a fine-tuned policy blueprint, but which provides the political satisfaction of actually having a chance of passage.

There is some evidence that today's reformers have taken this second lesson to heart (though simplicity and clarity still remain elusive). In announcing their reform intentions in 2007, all of the top-tier Democratic candidates for president—Senator Hillary Clinton, former Senator John Edwards, and Senator Barack Obama—eschewed both a "Medicare-For-All" plan and an individualized approach in which Americans would be required to obtain coverage outside of employment with the help of government subsidies and purchasing pools. Instead, they have embraced a messy mix of elements: (1) the creation of a new government insurance "menu" that would allow all Americans without workplace health insurance to choose among a range of regulated private health plans, as well as to enroll in a new public insurance plan modeled after Medicare; (2) a requirement that employers either provide coverage or pay a mandated contribution to help finance their workers' coverage through this new government pool (aka "play-or-pay"); and (3) a requirement—initially, or eventually if necessary—that all Americans show proof of coverage.

From a policy standpoint, this three-pronged approach lacks conceptual purity. But from a political standpoint, it has real virtues. For one, most workers who now enjoy good employer-provided insurance would continue, at least initially, to receive it at their place of work. For another, because employers would continue to play a major financing role, the federal costs and new taxes needed would be much lower than would be true under a Medicare-For-All plan or a universal individualized framework.

To provide a sense of these virtues, Lewin VHI recently estimated the impact of a health plan that I have developed with the support of the Economic Policy Institute, "Health Care for America." The proposal—a template for Clinton's, Edwards', and Obama's plans—requires employers to cover their workers or contribute 6 percent of payroll to the cost of workers' coverage. Workers whose employers make the contribution will be enrolled in a Medicare-like plan with generous benefits (they can, if desired, purchase regulated private insurance instead).

According to Lewin VHI's estimates, the proposal will cover all but a tiny sliver of the population younger than sixty-five—about half through the new federal system and half through employers. Yet it will actually reduce national health spending, cost the federal government a relatively modest $50 billion a year, and save states and employers substantial money. The reason the plan can cover everyone without driving up costs is that it capitalizes on Medicare's lower service prices, streamlined administration, and ability to get a better deal on drugs. Over time, moreover, this approach will dramatically reduce medical inflation, as public insurance is able to use its enhanced bargaining power to hold down costs.[35]

Finally, all these proposals embody a means of gradually moving away from America's embattled employment-based structure. If, as most expect, public insurance ends up proving capable of controlling costs better than employment-based plans (or if employers simply continue to retreat from coverage), then the public plan will over time come to enroll a larger share of Americans—without the massive disruption entailed by an overnight transformation. This is not an incidental feature of these proposals; it is the core of their strategy for gradually moving away from America's embedded employment-based structure.

But finding a policy design that will minimize public fears is, of course, only part of the battle. The bigger challenge is to build a coalition that can engage Americans constructively in the struggle while pressing their leaders to act. And that means coming to grips with the transformed political realities that stymied the Clinton plan.

THE NEW WORLD OF AMERICAN POLITICS

Largely unbeknownst to those who waged battle over President Clinton's proposal, the battle occurred amid — and, indeed, helped complete — a transition between two very different worlds of American politics.

The first world, already crumbling in the years leading up to Clinton's election, was one based on bipartisan compromise, often behind closed doors. It rested on the continuing sway of moderates, who in an era of divided government usually held the cards in high-stakes political fights. It was premised on some degree of insulation of the legislative process from special-interest arm-twisting and party strong-arming. And it required a broadly competitive electoral environment — the myriad fierce campaign fights every two years that ensured, as Reagan-era House Speaker Tip O'Neill famously put it, that "all politics is local."[36]

That world is gone, and it will not be returning soon. Congressional moderates are vanishing; campaign money and corporate lobbying hold greatly increased sway; and party leaders wield vastly more power than they did a generation ago. Even with the shift of Congress to the Democrats, competitive election contests remain few and far between. The result is greater party polarization — something long prized by political scientists enamored of parliamentary systems—but without the consistent electoral discipline that ensures that these polarized parties are accountable to middle-of-the-road voters. In Congress, the two parties are farther apart today than at any point in the last generation, mostly because of the movement of the Republican Party to the right since the 1970s. The motto of this new world was best summed up by Texas Republican Dick Armey, who helped lead the charge against the Clinton plan and then became House Majority Leader: "The first rule of politics is: Never offend your base."[37]

This motto played out vividly in 2008's campaign-driven health care debates. During the primary campaign, all the leading GOP contenders for president explicitly rejected large-scale reforms — and in particular any coverage requirement — even as all the leading Democratic candidates endorsed such changes. Even Reagan's evocative phrase "socialized medicine," which many thought had met its match when Medicare proved a popular success, returned to the heart of GOP rhetoric. Republicans from President Bush on down used the slogan in denouncing Democrats' attempts to expand publicly funded coverage for children through the State Children's Health Insurance Program (SCHIP). Meanwhile, in late 2007, GOP presidential contenders Rudy Giuliani and Mitt Romney lambasted the relatively cautious health proposals touted by the leading Democratic candidates as emulating "the socialist solution they have in Europe" (Giuliani) with the goal of imposing "a European-style socialized medicine plan" (Romney).

Indeed, many Republicans embraced a set of ideas barely discussed in the early 1990s and diametrically opposed to leading Democratic plans—subsidies for individually purchased insurance and Health Savings Accounts, as outlined by Quadagno and McKelvey in their chapter in this volume. In 1992, President George H. W. Bush put forth a substantial reform plan in response to the growing pressure for action. During the run-up to the 2008 election, no one had any expectation that President George W. Bush—whose major health policy move in 2007 was his successive vetoing of congressional Democrats' attempts to expand SCHIP—would do the same.

Back in 1993 and 1994, the Clinton health policy team seemed flummoxed by the shifting sands they stepped onto. Torn between the old politics and the new, they embraced a cause that cheered the Democratic base, then adopted a proposal that alienated much of it; packed their proposal with special favors for organized labor, then campaigned against organized labor to create the North American Free Trade Agreement (NAFTA); expected liberal committee chairs to play their game even as they made clear that congressional moderates were their lodestar. Behind the back-and-forth darting was the assumption that, at some point, somehow, a bipartisan deal would be forged in the back room, as it had been on tax reform in 1986 and Social Security in 1983. But the political preconditions for such a bargain were gone—swept away by growing partisan warfare.

This time, it is clear that the fight will take place on the scorched earth left by these battles. And this means that the fight will require updated strategies: greater willingness to compromise on means yet greater clarity on ends, an attention to coalition building from the very beginning, and hard thinking about procedural reforms that could reduce minority obstruction, including the threat of a Senate filibuster — the major barrier to change within Congress, now that the filibuster has become an all-purpose tool of minority party obstruction. It will also require serious efforts to bring on board committed reformers who support a universal Medicare plan, and to provide them with the guarantees and arguments they need to embrace a less inspiring but more politically palatable approach. Here, a true commitment to a public insurance option, offered on a level playing field with regulated private plans, could prove crucial.

Given all this, universal health insurance looks likely to happen in the near term — or rather more likely to happen, since the odds are long regardless — only if a Democrat occupies the White House. But even if a Democrat were to occupy the Oval Office and Democrats augmented their standing in Congress in 2008, as most political analysts expect, there remains the difficult task of building a reform coalition in Congress and beyond. In 1993, President Bill Clinton pursued a strategy that ended up alienating both congressional liberals and congressional conservatives. In 2009, any Democratic president will have to do better to have any chance of success.

The main challenge is not to develop an even more detailed health plan, which could and should be left to Congress. In 1993, in part because President Clinton received advice to this effect from congressional Democratic leaders, the Clinton administration set up a massive internal process to refine the plan that had been decided upon during the campaign, a process that took up valuable time and short-circuited congressional and interest-group bargaining. Decades of research on presidential power suggest the limits of presidential policy fine-tuning in the domestic arena. Whatever Democratic leaders say, a new Democratic president should follow the path that President Bush successfully blazed on tax cuts in 2001: develop the broad outlines, then leave it to Congress to broker the deals. But the challenges will still be enormous: to bring advocates of action together around a reform vision that can attract moderate backing, and then to cross-pressure those moderates by mobilizing the support of the public and important allied groups.

Alongside the looming obstacles, there are promising signs for change. Galvanized by the Bush presidency and linked by the Internet, progressive activists have gained some of the passion and grassroots power that was once seen only on the conservative side. Organized labor is displaying both greater boldness and greater pragmatism. There may be room to run with key segments of the business community, as corporate leaders increasingly realize they are caught between the rock of rising costs and the hard place of hurting workers. And workers clearly are hurting, as medical costs escalate and private insurance declines.

The great unanswered question is whether a public disillusioned about politics can be brought to kindle some faith in their leaders and their government. Americans say they believe in government action to universalize health insurance.[38] They say they want reform to be a top priority. Similar sentiments helped bring health care to the top of the agenda in the early 1990s, and reformers are on the verge of having their moment in the sun again. With the lessons of the past in mind, and fortune on their side, perhaps they can finally seize it.

NOTES

1   Max J. Skidmore, "Ronald Reagan and 'Operation Coffeecup': A Hidden Episode in American Political History," *Journal of American Culture* 12, no. 3 (1989): 89–96.

2   See James Farr, Jacob S. Hacker, and Nicole Kazee, "The Policy Scientist of Democracy: The Discipline of Harold Lasswell," *American Political Science Review* 100, no. 4 (2006): 579–87; and Farr, Hacker, and Kazee, "Revisiting Lasswell," *Policy Sciences* 41, no. 1 (2008): 21–32.

3   This section draws on Jacob S. Hacker, "Dismantling the Health Care State? Political Institutions, Public Policies, and the Comparative Politics of Health Reform," *British Journal of Political Science* 34 (2004): 693–724.

4   Joseph White, *Competing Solutions: American Health Care Proposals and International Experience* (Washington, DC: Brookings Institution, 1995).

5   See Evelyne Huber and John Stephens, *Development and Crisis of the Welfare State: Parties and Politics in Global Markets* (Chicago: University of Chicago Press, 2001). Using Huber and Stephens's dataset (http://www.lisproject.org/publications/welfaredata) and OECD expenditure data, the correlation between 1945–75 cumulative left-party governance and the 1975 private share of health spending is -0.58.

6   In the OECD, only Italy's national health service was not enacted under social democratic rule.

7   Ellen Immergut, *Health Politics: Interests and Institutions in Western Europe* (New York: Cambridge University Press, 1992).

8   See, for example, Sven Steinmo and Jon Watts, "It's the Institutions, Stupid! Why Comprehensive National Health Insurance Always Fails in America," *Journal of Health Politics, Policy and Law* 20, no. 2 (1995): 329–72.

9   Jacob S. Hacker, "The Historical Logic of National Health Insurance: Structure and Sequence in the Development of British, Canadian, and U.S. Medical Policy," *Studies in American Political Development* 12, no. 2 (Spring 1998): 57–130.

10 Paul Pierson, "Increasing Returns, Path Dependence, and the Study of Politics," *American Political Science Review* 94 (2000): 251–67.

11 Jacob S. Hacker, *The Divided Welfare State: The Battle over Public and Private Social Benefits in the United States* (New York: Cambridge University Press, 2002).

12 Frank D. Campion, *The AMA and U.S. Health Policy since 1940* (Chicago: Chicago Review Press, 1984), 162.

13 "Memorandum of the Congress of Industrial Organizations in Support of the Principle that Employer Payments for the Cost of Group Hospitalization Medical and Like Benefits are not Taxable Income to the Employee," Office of Tax Policy, Box 4, National Archives and Records Administration, 1.

14 Ibid., 19.

15 Ibid., 22. The 1949 quote is from the testimony of James B. Carey to Subcommittee on Health of the Committee on Labor and Public Welfare, *National Health Program, 1949* (Washington, DC: U.S. GPO, 1949), 421.

16 Paul Starr to Ira Magaziner, memorandum, 22 Mar. 1993; quoted in Jacob S. Hacker, *The Road to Nowhere: The Genesis of President Clinton's Plan for Health Security* (Princeton, NJ: Princeton University Press, 1997), 128.

17 Paul Starr and Walter L. Zelman, "A Bridge to Compromise: Competition Under a Budget," *Health Affairs* 12, Supplement 1 (1993): 7–23.

18 Robert Patricelli, Chamber of Commerce, to Ira Magaziner, May 10, 1993; quoted in Hacker, *The Road to Nowhere*, 135.

19 Walter Zelman to Bob Boorstin, March 10, 1993; quoted in Hacker, *Road to Nowhere*, 136.

20 *Consumer Reports*, "Health Insurance Survey Reveals 1 in 4 People Insured but Not Adequately Covered," September 2007.

21 The Kaiser Family Foundation, *Employer Health Benefits, 2007 Summary of Findings*, http://www.kff.org/insurance/7672/upload/Summary-of-Findings-EHBS-2007 .pdf; and Jared Bernstein and Heidi Shierholz, "A Decade of Decline: The Erosion of Employer-Provided Health Care in the United States and California, 1995–

2006," *EPI Briefing Paper #209,* April 16, 2008.

22 The Kaiser Family Foundation, *Employer Health Benefits, 2007.*

23 Cristina Boccuti and Marilyn Moon, "Comparing Medicare and Private Insurers: Growth Rates in Spending over Three Decades," *Health Affairs* 22, no. 2 (2003): 230–37.

24 Gerard F. Anderson, Uwe E. Reinhardt, Peter S. Hussey and Varduhi Petroysan, "It's the Prices, Stupid: Why the United States Is So Different from Other Countries," *Health Affairs* 22, no. 3 (2003): 89–105.

25 McKinsey & Company, "Accounting for the Cost of Health Care in the U.S.," January 2007, http://www.mckinsey.com/mgi/reports/pdfs/healthcare/MGI_US_HC_ fullreport.pdf.

26 Karen Davis, Cathy Schoen, Stephen C. Schoenbaum, Michelle M. Doty, Alyssa L. Holmgren, Jennifer L. Kriss, and Katherine K. Shea, "Mirror, Mirror on the Wall: An International Update on the Comparative Performance of American Health Care," 59 (The Commonwealth Fund, May 15, 2007).

27 Ellen Nolte and C. Martin McKee, "Measuring the Health of Nations: Updating an Earlier Analysis," *Health Affairs* 27, no. 1 (2008): 58–71.

28 This conclusion has been popularized by Drew Westen, *The Political Brain: The Role of Emotion in Deciding the Fate of the Nation* (New York: Public Affairs Books, 2007).

29 New York Times/CBS News Poll, February 23–27, 2007, http://graphics8.nytimes .com/packages/pdf/national/03022007_poll.pdf.

30 Jeffrey Jones, "Low Trust in Federal Government Rivals Watergate Era Levels," *Gallup News,* September 26, 2007; and Joseph Nye, Philip Zelikow, and David King, eds., *Why People Don't Trust Government* (Cambridge, MA: Harvard University Press, 1997).

31 For a good recent compendium of polls, see Ruy Teixeira, "What the Public Really Wants on Health Care," The Century Foundation, December 4, 2006, http://tcf.org/ publications/healthcare/wtprw.healthcare.pdf. See also, Kaiser Family Foundation/ Harvard School of Public Health, "The Public's Health Care Agenda for the New Congress and Presidential Campaign," December 2006, http://www.kff.org/ kaiserpolls/upload/7597.pdf.

32 Most striking is the increasing liberalism seen in James Stimson's "public mood" series, which uses multiple survey questions asked with the same wording over time to track the liberalism or conservatism of the American public. Stimson's data show that in 2004, the public mood was more liberal than at any point since 1961. Updated from James A. Stimson, *Public Opinion in America: Moods, Cycles,*

and Swings, 2nd ed. (Boulder, CO: Westview Press, 1999), http://www.unc.edu/~jstimson/time.html.

33 Ylan Q. Mui and Dale Russakoff, "Wal-Mart, Union Join Forces on Health Care; Alliance's Goal Is to Improve Coverage," *Washington Post,* 8 February 2007, D1.

34 In a February 2007 poll, for example, 64 percent of respondents agreed that "the federal government should guarantee health insurance for all Americans," while 27 percent disagreed. Asked to choose between universal coverage and maintaining recent tax cuts, 76 percent chose universal coverage; 60 percent said they would be willing to pay higher taxes to cover the uninsured. New York Times/CBS News Poll, 23–27 February 2007, http://graphics8.nytimes.com/packages/pdf/national/03022007_poll.pdf.

35 Jacob S. Hacker, "Health Care for America: A Proposal for Guaranteed, Affordable Health Care for All Americans Building on Medicare and Employment-Based Insurance," *Economic Policy Institute Briefing Paper* No. 180, January 11, 2007, http://www.sharedprosperity.org/bp180.html. These estimates were done by Lewin VHI.

36 Tip O' Neill and Gary Hymel, *All Politics Is Local: And Other Rules of the Game* (New York: Crown, 1993).

37 Quoted in Jacob S. Hacker and Paul Pierson, *Off Center: The Republican Revolution and the Erosion of American Democracy* (New Haven, CT: Yale University Press, 2005), 110.

38 In December 2007, 65 percent of Americans supported a "universal health insurance program in which everyone is covered under a program like Medicare that is run by the government and financed by taxpayers." Associated Press–Yahoo Poll, December 14–20, 2007, http://news.yahoo.com/page/election-2008-political-pulse-voter-worries. Even greater enthusiasm can be found for a play-or-pay requirement: nearly nine of ten Democrats and four of five independents, and even 73 percent of Republicans, express support. Commonwealth Fund Biennial Health Insurance Survey, June–October 2007, www.commonwealthfund.org/publications/publications_show.htm?doc_id=647816.

Contributors

JACOB S. HACKER is professor of political science at the University of California at Berkeley, where he codirects the Center on Health and Economic Security at the Boalt Law School. A frequent media commentator and author of numerous scholarly and popular articles, he is the author of four books, most recently *The Great Risk Shift: The New Economic Insecurity and the Decline of the American Dream* and *Off Center: The Republican Revolution and the Erosion of American Democracy* (coauthored with Paul Pierson).

ELIZABETH A. MCGLYNN is an associate director for RAND Health and holds the RAND Distinguished Chair in Health Care Quality. Dr. McGlynn is an internationally known expert on methods for assessing and reporting on quality of health care delivery. She is leading RAND Health's COMPARE initiative, which is developing a comprehensive method for evaluating health reform proposals. Dr. McGlynn is a member of the Institute of Medicine and serves on several national advisory committees.

J. BRANDON MCKELVEY is a doctoral student and Presidential Fellow in sociology at Florida State University. He has authored and coauthored articles on the privatization of health care and changing workplace expectations for aging workers due to globalization.

DAVID MELTZER is associate professor of medicine, economics, and public policy at the University of Chicago, where he is chief of the Section of Hospital Medicine and director of the Center for Health and the Social Sciences. His research examines a variety of areas in health economics, including the theoretical foundations of medical cost-effectiveness and the cost and quality of hospital care.

JILL QUADAGNO is professor of sociology at Florida State University where she holds the Mildred and Claude Pepper Eminent Scholar Chair in Social Gerontology. She is past president of the American Sociological Association and served as senior policy advisor on the President's Bi-Partisan Commission on Entitlement and Tax Reform. She is the author of 12 books and more than 50 articles on aging and social policy issues. Her most recent book is *One Nation: Uninsured: Why the U.S. Has No National Health Insurance.*

KATHERINE SWARTZ is professor of health economics and policy at Harvard School of Public Health. She is a member of the Institute of Medicine and author of *Reinsuring Health: Why More Middle-Class People Are Uninsured and What Government Can Do.* From 1995 to 2007, Professor Swartz was editor of *Inquiry,* a journal that focuses on health care organization, provision, and financing. Between November 2008 and November 2009, she will be the president of the Association of Public Policy Analysis and Management (APPAM).

DEBORAH THORNE is assistant professor of sociology at Ohio University and a principal investigator on the Consumer Bankruptcy Project. For the past decade, consumer bankruptcy has been at the core of her research agenda. As such, she has authored articles on various issues associated with consumer bankruptcy such as social mobility, stigma, gender, and medical debt.

ELIZABETH WARREN is the Leo Gottlieb Professor of Law at Harvard University. She has written eight books and more than a hundred scholarly articles dealing with credit and economic stress. Her latest two books are *The Two-Income Trap* and *All Your Worth.* Warren was the chief adviser to the National Bankruptcy Review Commission and she currently serves as a member of the Commission on Economic Inclusion established by the FDIC.